# PALEO SLOW COOKER

**You Wondering What You Can Cook Using Your Slow Cooker?
Learn The Best Way To Maximize Your Slow Cooker?
Lose Weight by the Best Diet and Feel Stronger**

**Most of people these days chose to cook with slow cooker. Its main benefit is that it saves time, save money and energy. You can put all the ingredients in, set the slow cooker and leave for work. When you come from work you can have a delicious, healthy warm dinner at home.
This is a 2 books that give you:**

## 1. PALEO DIET-FOR BEGINNERS And
## 2. SLOW COOKER COOKBOOK

**You will get the best Diet and Make the most use of your Slow Cooker
The Beginners Guide to Paleo Diet and Its Best Recipes
Recipes from Breakfast, Lunches and Dinner
Quick and Easy Healthy Food Recipes
Best Method of Food Preparation
Clear Instruction with step by step And So Much More!**

## Table of Contents

# PALEO DIET FOR BEGINNERS

*THE ESSENTIALS GUIDE TO PALEO DIET
THAT HELPS YOU TO LOSE WEIGHT,
BUILD MUSCLE AND LIVE HEALTHIER*

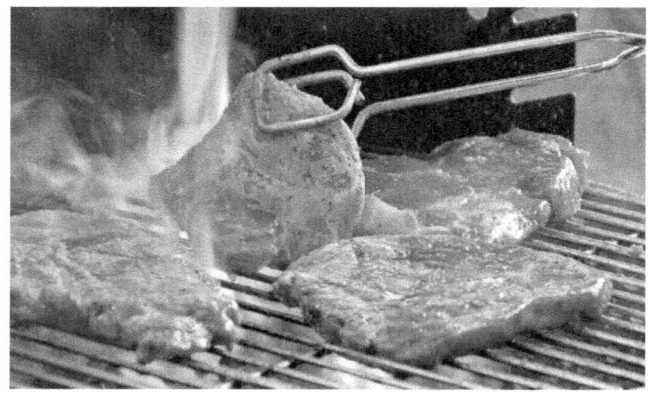

**MARIA COOK**

# COPYRIGHT

This document is geared towards providing exact and reliable information in regards to the topic and issue covered. The publication is sold with the idea that the publisher is not required to render accounting, officially permitted, or otherwise, qualified services. If advice is necessary, legal or professional, a practiced individual in the profession should be ordered.

- From a Declaration of Principles which was accepted and approved equally by a Committee of the American Bar Association and a Committee of Publishers and Associations.

The information provided in this book is for educational and entertainment purposes only. The author is not a physician and this is not to be taken as medical advice or a recommendation to stop taking medications. The information provided in this book is based on the author's experiences and interpretations of the past and current research available. You should consult your physician to insure the daily habits and principles in this book are appropriate for your individual circumstances. If you have any health issues or pre-existing conditions, please consult your doctor before implementing any of the information you have learned in this book. Results will vary from individual to individual. This book is for informational purposes only and the author does not accept any responsibilities for any liabilities or damages, real or perceived, resulting from the use of this information.

The information herein is offered for informational purposes solely, and is universal as so. The presentation of the information is without contract or any type of guarantee assurance.

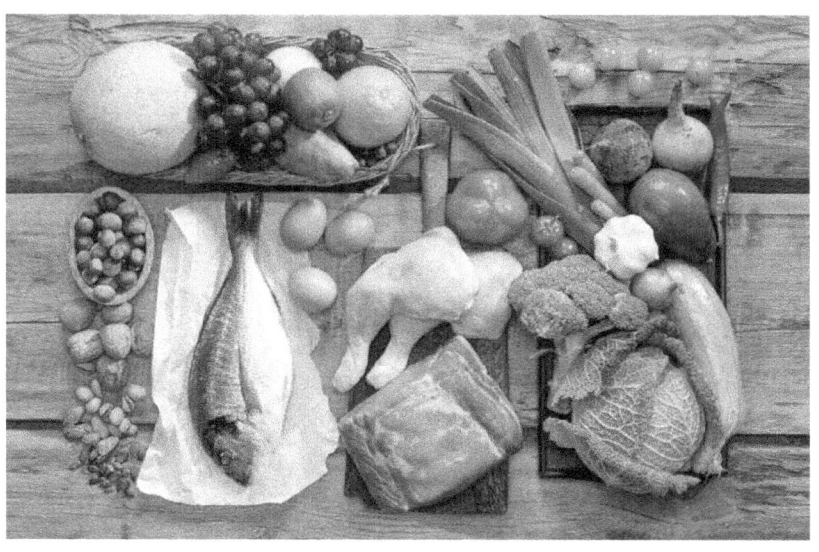

# INTRODUCTION

For over 50 years 'dietary professionals' have been telling us what to eat and drink. They've told us to consume lots of grains and carbohydrates, drink milk, avoid cholesterol, stay away from red meat and run screaming at the sight of fat. The result? For over 50 years our waistlines have expanded, with obesity growing from 12% of the population back then to 35% today. You can see it in your neighborhood, with people ballooning year by year. Kids are so overweight they can't play tag anymore. Middle-aged people need walking frames because their bones can't support their weight. And most people's medicine cabinet's look like somebody in the house has got cancer.

Something has gone terribly wrong.

The government has admitted as much. Recently, they've announced they're dropped the low-fat diet as well as their guidelines for avoiding cholesterol. These changes came after it became clear that Harvard's clinical trials could not replicate the research findings on which many of the dietary guidelines are based.

The question then becomes, if not that diet which one then? Obviously, if they've been misguiding us for the ever so many years, then we need to return to an older, more honest way of living. A way that we've evolved to follow and which naturally suits our bodies. We should, in other words, return to the Paleo Diet.

Our prehistoric ancestors ate and lived very differently. The result was that they lived longer and their lives were healthier. So if we can return to a lifestyle more in line with how they lived, our lives will improve as well. We'll have more energy, live more honestly, be sick less often, reduce our weight and bring ourselves in line with how we're supposed to live. Our lives will return to something as close to natural as is possible in this modern-day world.

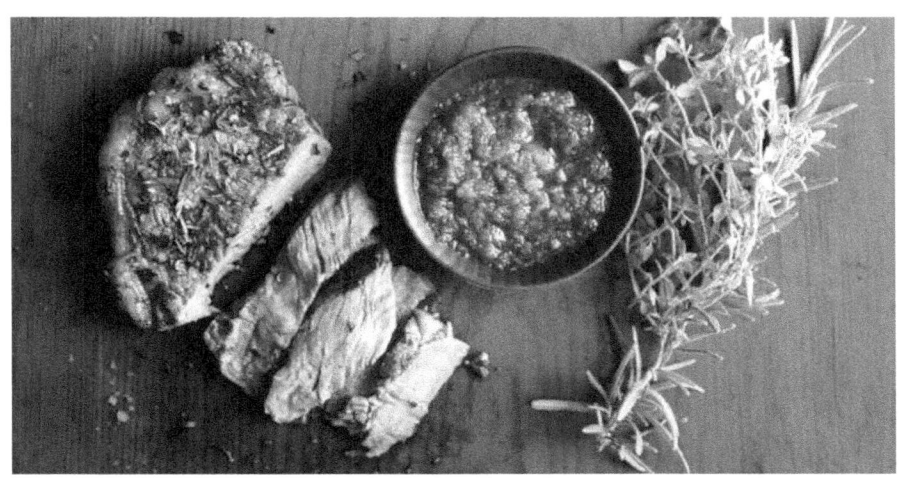

Unlike most fad diets, the Paleo diet is a sustainable, long-term diet. It regulates hormonal balance and positive gene expression. This leads to better health and well-being, enhanced athletic performance and body composition. The Paleo diet is a one of the most widely supported diets in the world. Celebrities, clinical experts and dietitians recommend it as the best way to restore balance, fight medical conditions and reduce the waistline.

Also known as the caveman diet, the stone-age diet or hunter-gatherer diet, the Paleo Diet is low in carbohydrates, while being high in protein and fat. It focuses on the consumption of fruits, vegetables and nuts and rejects processed and man-made foods. The diet's central premise is that humanity has not changed much since our hunter-gatherer past. Thus we should shift away from modern culinary inventions. Instead we should focus on eating the way we did back then in order for us to live longer and healthier lives.

It was originally conceived by Walter L. Voegtlin, a famous gastroenterologist, in the 1970s. His version was meat-based and contained few carbohydrates. The diet gained mainstream attention in the 1980s through the work of Melvin Konner and S. Boyd Eaton. They modified it so that it included some foods not available to hunter-gatherers, like whole-grain bread.

Whatever the name or the specific guidelines, you can't deny the diet's benefits. Millions swear by it, convinced it has changed their lives for the better. It's not just them. Every year, new studies supporting their claims that it has physical and psychological health benefit are published.

So what are you waiting for? Don't live a junk life, don't choose for junk food. Instead, opt for a healthier way of life, choose less stress, choose reduced depression, and choose less medicine. Choose Paleo.

Before engaging in a new diet consult a doctor or a dietician

Please be aware that changing your diet to a Paleo Diet is a serious undertaking, which will change what you eat and how you live life. It should not be undertaken without careful consideration. Before starting on the diet, speak to your doctor or a dietitian, especially if you've got a preexisting medical condition.

# GOING PALEO WAY

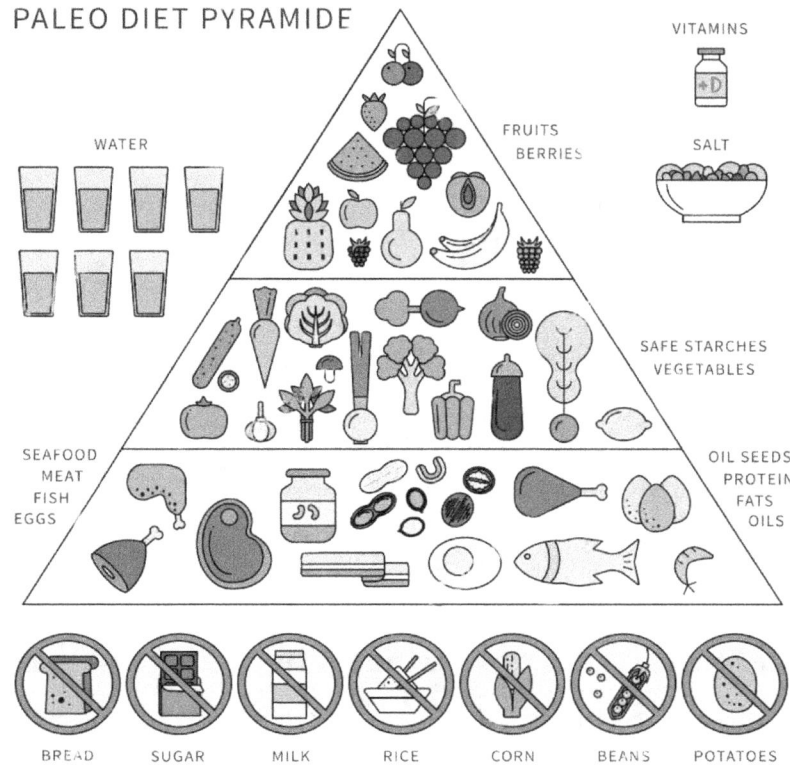

To go Paleo you need to avoid grains, potatoes, legumes, dairy, refined and processed products, certain vegetable oils, and refined sugar. Instead, focus on fish, grass-fed meats, fruits, and vegetables. Fresh organic produce from a local source is even better. Unlike what you may have heard, the Paleo Diet is not a strict raw-food diet and food can be eaten either raw or cooked. Practitioners encourage a great deal of variety in the diet to ensure the proper balance of vitamins and minerals.

The health benefits of the diet are many. It will:

- Reduce the quantities of stored fat, thereby causing weight loss and toning.

- Fill you up with antioxidants, phytonutrients and other vitamins through the large amount of fruit you'll be consuming.

- Reduce your risk for cancer and heart disease.

- Reduce and bring under control type II diabetes. It does this in two ways. First, it improves your glucose tolerance, decreases insulin secretion and increases insulin sensitivity. Second, it eliminates foods such as grains or refined sugars.

- Lead to muscle gain, better digestion, less stress, more energy, better sleep, reduced aging, smoother skin, stronger bones, healthier teeth, a stronger immune system and higher fertility.

- Help with celiac disease, heart disease, Crohn's disease, IBS, IBD, heart burn, leaky gut, ulcers, allergies, and asthma.

- Improve brain function, by way of providing essential vitamins and proteins such as omega 3, due to the diet's high quantity of fresh fish. Omega 3 fatty acids are essential for brain development and healthy eyes and heart.

What you won't need to do with this diet is count your calories, or control your portions (Do you think prehistoric man ever counted their calories?). Instead, this diet relies solely on the foods that you eat to induce these health benefits.

# HOW PALEO WORKS

- You simply take out all of the processed food that early man never ate. Yes, all of it. Dairy, refined sugar, chemicals, processed food. You clean your body of all the unnecessary fuel that is storing itself on your hips and heart as fat. Many modern diseases can be prevented by simply eating healthily, so why complicate your life?

- Paleo is all about natural food. You eliminate the overly-processed supermarket meals and gain your energy from healthy food, the sun and wind and freedom. Sounds romantic? It is. Let's start with what to avoid, so you can be joyful later.

## What to Avoid

Artificial sweeteners and any added sugars: This includes stevia, agave, molasses, aspartame, brown sugar, high fructose corn syrup, maple syrup, and sucralose just to mention a few

Legumes: This includes white beans, garbanzo beans, red beans, black beans, pinto beans and lentils

Vegetable oils that are high in omega 6: These include peanut oil, palm kernel oil, canola oil, corn and soy, cottonseed, safflower, sunflower etc.

Grains: These include wheat, rye, buckwheat, oats, sorghum, corn, wild rice and quinoa just to mention a few.


Just to give you some motivation to go the paleo way, here are some benefits that you are likely to derive if you go paleo.

*It gives you a healthy brain*

Coldwater fish is one of the best sources of proteins and fat. This is one of the foods you can eat while on a paleo diet. The preferred cold water fish is a wild caught salmon. Its fat is full of omega 3 fatty acids, which contain DHA, which is perfect for the eyes and more importantly for the development of your brain.

*Enough vitamins and minerals*

Vegetables are a major food group in the Paleo diet. You get to eat the rainbow i.e. the different colors of all the veggies, which suggest the different nutrients they contain.

*You gain more of muscle and less of fat*

The Paleo diet relies on meat, which contains a great dose of healthy proteins. The protein is useful in development of new cells.

*Your gut becomes healthier*

Manmade fats, sugar, and all other processed junk affect your intestines negatively. They cause inflammation on your gut and give you the 'leaky gut syndrome'. The Paleo diet doesn't allow consumption of any of these products, which means that you are likely to have a healthier gut.

*Better absorption of food and digestion*

You get to eat food that your body is adapted to from way back, which simply means that the body is likely to digest and absorb it perfectly.

*Dropping a few pounds*

The Paleo diet is low on carbohydrates. Obviously, carbohydrates contribute greatly to weight gain. Therefore, the Paleo diet will in turn fuel great weight loss for you. The diet also advocates for the consumption of more green vegetables. These are rich in fiber, which can keep you full for longer, which can in turn ensure that you don't end up feeling hungry thus yielding to the temptation to snack or binge. This in turn means that you will end up eating fewer calories thus pushing your body into a calorie deficit situation that in turn makes the body burn stored fats for energy.

- **Sugar** - It goes without saying that refined sugar is harmful and not just for our teeth. From the moment sugar gets into your stomach, it starts transforming into glucose. 20,000 years ago, that would have been extremely helpful in keeping us running after deer over miles and miles of forests, hills and meadows. In our more sedentary society, all that glucose gets stuck on our hips and belly even worse than eating fat would. Refined sugar is even more dangerous, as the industrial process makes it extra-sweet, turning it into an internal time bomb of an overload of calories and damaging your cells. Not to mention the risk of diabetes.

- **Dairy** - Being on dairy-free diet can greatly improve your energy levels. Our stomachs are not designed to digest milk. Some of us develop a lactose intolerance which makes life no fun at all. But in social settings it's hard to avoid cakes and other desserts that are made with butter, cheese, cream and milk. But we give you 6 amazing desserts that are delicious and you'll never miss the dairy or refined sugar. Paleo replacements are easy find.

- **Grains** - Any bread, pasta and crackers. And anything remotely tied to wheat and most other grains. Grains are made of carbs and turn themselves into glucose in your body. This would be ok, if you were still running over hills every minute of every day. All that extra glucose is stored as fat, because it's not needed. Bread is hard to give, but once you break through, there'll be no turning back. A gluten free diet is the only known cure for celiac disease, which affects the small intestine in pretty painful ways.

## What is better?

Remember what we said about Paleo lifestyle not starving you, but feeding you? Yes, it's true, this is the healthiest way to lose weight you'll ever find. You are cleaning your body of extra fat simply by refusing to ingest any more refined sugar and industrially over processed substances. When you stop eating useless food, you'll not only feel more rested, but also a lot fresher, like breathing in mountain air in the morning. And you won't go hungry. Paleo recipes are nourishing and low in calories.

## What to Eat:

Nuts and Seeds: Walnuts, pecans, pumpkin seeds, pine nuts, macadamia nuts, almonds, hazelnuts, cashews etc.

Meat and Fish: Lamb, pork, beef, chicken (poultry), turkey, buffalo, tuna, shrimp, lobster, trout, salmon, halibut, sardines, tilapia, mackerel, clams etc.

Beverages: Filtered water, vegetable juice, fruit juice, herbal tea etc.

Fats and Oils: Walnut oil, avocado oil, macadamia oil, hazelnut oil, tallow, lard, coconut oil, extra virgin olive oil etc.

Vegetables and Fruits: Berries (blueberries, strawberries, blackberries, cranberries etc.), banana, apricot, apple, guava, cantaloupe, lemon, papaya, mango, orange, kiwi, honeydew, peaches, melons, tomato, watercress, zucchini, tangerine, pumpkin, Swiss chard, squash, spinach, turnips, peppers, onions, kales, eggplant, mustard, Brussels sprouts, broccoli, celery, beets, asparagus, artichokes, carrots, dandelion, mushrooms etc.

Here are the main points:

- Meat – non-processed, of course. The more organic, the better.

- Fish – now you have an excuse to go fishing

- Birds

- Eggs

- Natural oils – coconut oil, olive oil, etc.

- Good carbs – the good cop is here and you'll find it in vegetables and sweet potatoes

- Fruits

- Vegetables

- Seeds, Nuts

- Honey

- Potatoes – sweet potatoes are the best

## Lose the Weight

- The Paleo diet is the best diet for losing weight, because it relies on you're not feeling hungry. All of this food is nourishing and will keep you satisfied for hours.

## The Guidelines

1. Enjoy protein with every meal.

2. Go overboard with the fruits and vegetables; either cooked or raw!

3. As far as meat and fish are concerned, buy organic or free range if your budget allows. No hormones or chemicals. Low in saturated fat.

4. Be reasonable with your use of salt, use sea salt. Remember that many condiments are loaded with chemicals, additives, sodium, so look for organic condiments and read the ingredient list or make your own.

5. Exercise, this will increase your feeling of well-being from the natural hormones that your body produces when you exercise and you'll be able to take advantage of all the extra energy you are going to have!

6. Little or no saturated fats - avocado works great in many instances. One of my favorite breakfasts is scrabbled egg whites along with gluten free toast with seeds, a little extra virgin olive oil, avocado, sea salt, freshly ground black pepper and some red chili flakes.

7. Limit your consumption of alcohol. Choose good quality wine and stay away from cocktails laden with sugar and artificial ingredients.

Here are some of the Paleo Recipes to get started

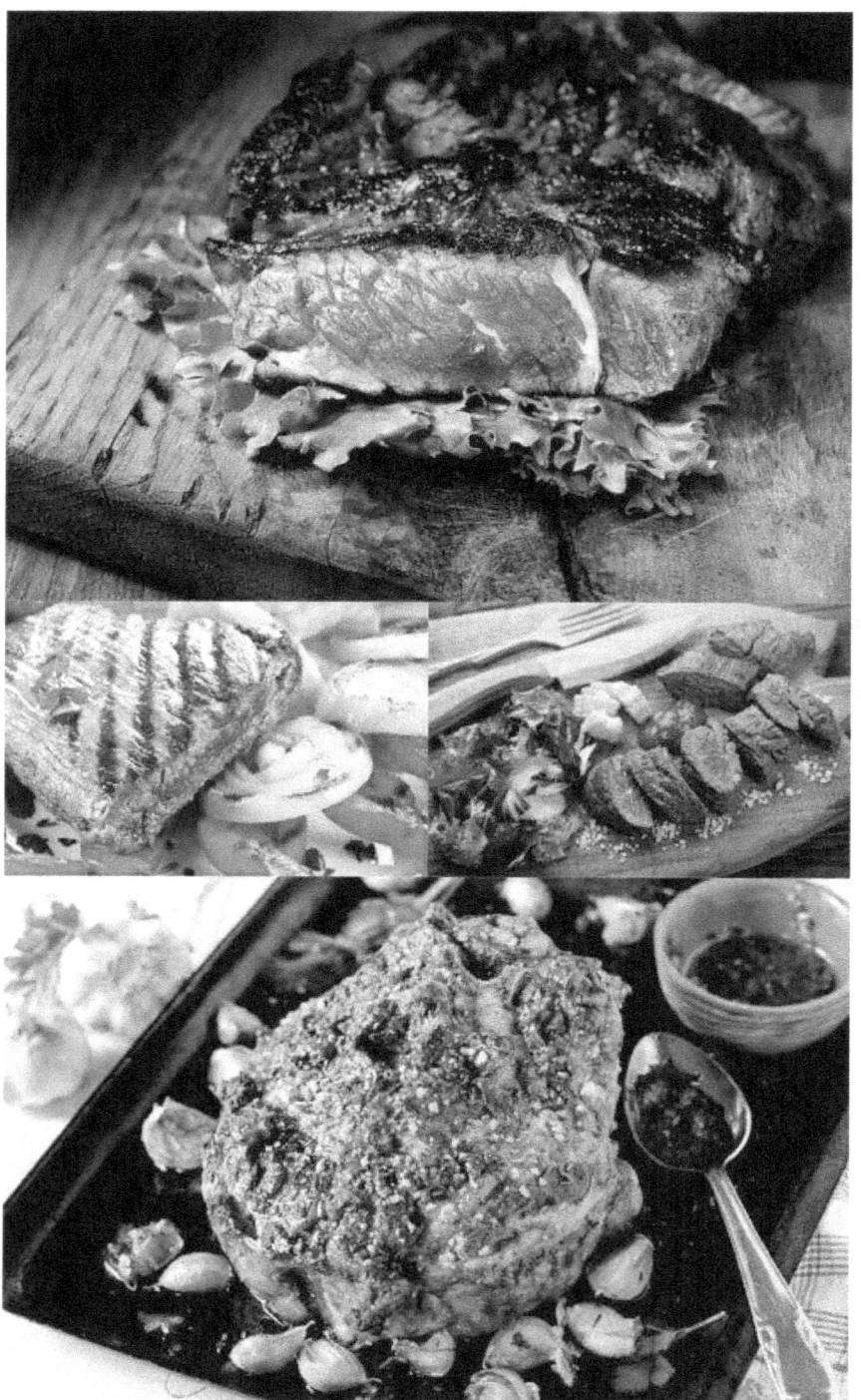

# BREAKFAST RECIPES

## Chunky Chili Breakfast Wrap

Serves: 4

Prep Time: 20 mins

**Ingredients**

- 1 pound lean ground beef

- 1 carrot, peeled, diced

- 1 medium onion, diced

- 1 celery stalk, diced

- 2 tomatoes, diced

- 1/2 cup water

- 4 cloves garlic, minced

- 1 tsp. oregano, cumin, paprika

- 1 tsp. salt, coarse black pepper

- Extra virgin olive oil

- 4 flax tortillas

## Directions

1.   Lightly coat 4 qt. slow cooker with olive oil.

2.   Place all ingredients in slow cooker and cook on low overnight for eight hours.

3.   In the morning, spoon chili into tortillas, roll and enjoy.

## Nutrition

- Calories 242

- Carbs 10

- Fat 13

- Protein 30

- Sodium 141

## Breakfast Bacon Bite Wraps

Serves: 4

Prep Time: 10 mins.

## Ingredients

- 8 slices bacon

- 2 cucumbers

- 4 eggs, hard boiled

- 1/2 tsp. salt, black pepper

## Directions

1. Peel eggs and mix in food processor until fairly smooth.

2. Heat skillet and cook bacon slices for three minutes per side.

3. Using mandolin, slice cucumbers into long pliable strips.

4. Place one slice cucumber on flat surface, half slice of bacon, dollop of egg and roll like sushi.

5. Repeat with remaining ingredients.

## Nutrition

- Calories 292

- Carbs 6

- Fat 20

- Protein 21

- Sodium 942

## Creamy Avocado Egg Salad Wrap

Serves: 4

Prep Time: 10 mins.

**Ingredients**

- 4 eggs, hard boiled

- 1 red bell pepper, seeded and chopped

- 1 celery stalk, chopped

- 1/2 avocado

- 1 lemon, juiced

- 1/2 tsp. salt, black pepper

- 4 almond wraps

**Directions**

1.    Peel eggs, chop and mix with celery, bell pepper in glass bowl.

2.    Place avocado in blender and mix until smooth, add lemon juice, salt, pepper.

3. Add avocado to bowl and mix.

4. Place a quarter of mixture in each wrap.

## Nutrition

- Calories 124

- Carbs 4

- Fat 9

- Protein 6

- Sodium 68

## Cashew Butter Banana Wrap

Serves: 4

Prep Time: 10 mins.

## Ingredients

- 1 cup cashews, soaked overnight

- 3 tbsp. sesame oil

- ¼ tsp. salt

- 2 bananas, peeled and sliced

- 4 flax wraps

## Directions

1.    Place cashews, sesame oil, salt in food processor and mix, scrape sides of bowl intermittently to ensure smooth mixture.

2.    Spread each wrap with cashew butter, add banana and wrap it up for breakfast.

## Nutrition

- Calories 339

- Carbs 24

- Fat 26

- Protein 6

- Sodium 153

# Smoked Salmon Eggs Wrap

Serves: 4

Prep Time: 10 mins.

## Ingredients

- 4 slices smoked salmon

- 6 eggs

- ¼ cup radish, shredded

- 1 lemon, juiced

- ½ tsp. salt, pepper

- 4 almond wraps

## Directions

1.  Mix radish with lemon juice, set aside.

2.  Whisk eggs with salt, pepper.

3.  Heat 2 tbsp. extra virgin olive oil in nonstick pan.

4.  Pour eggs into pan and cook a minute per side.

5.  Divide omelet into four sections.

6.  Place a quarter of omelet on almond wrap, top with smoked salmon and shredded radish and roll.

## Nutrition

- Calories 217

- Carbs 6

- Fat 7

- Protein 27

- Sodium 269

# LUNCH RECIPES

## Gourmet Chicken Caesar Wrap

Serves: 4

Prep Time: 15 mins.

**Ingredients**

- 1 lb. chicken breasts

- 3 tbsp. sardines, chopped

- 1 egg

- 1 tsp. dry mustard

- ½ lemon, juiced

- 2 cups green leaf lettuce, chopped

- ½ tsp. salt, black pepper

- Extra virgin olive oil

## Directions

1.  Preheat oven to 375 degrees and lightly coat glass baking dish with olive oil.

2.  Combine sardines, egg, dry mustard, lemon juice, salt and pepper in food processor and mix until creamy.

3.  Place chicken breasts in bottom of glass baking dish and pour creamy sauce over top.

4.  Bake in oven for 20 minutes turning halfway.

5.  Slice chicken breasts into strips, place on wrap alongside lettuce and wrap.

## Nutrition

- Calories 246

- Carbs 0

- Fat 10

- Protein 35

- Sodium 148

# Thai Lime Pork Wraps

Serves: 4

Prep Time: 10 mins

## Ingredients

- 1 lb. pork tenderloin

- 1 onion, sliced

- 2 limes, juiced

- 1 tsp. salt, black pepper

- 8 large lettuce leaves

- Extra virgin olive oil

## Directions

1.    Preheat oven to 400 degrees, lightly coat baking tray with extra virgin olive oil.

2.    Slice tenderloin into 1" pieces and toss with lime juice, salt pepper.

3.    Place tenderloin into oven to cook for 30 minutes.

4.    Place lettuce leaves on flat surface, spoon a little tenderloin per lettuce leaf, top with onion slices, roll and secure with toothpick.

# Sweet Potato Burrito Caramelized Onions

Serves: 4

Prep Time: 15 mins.

## Ingredients

- 2 sweet potatoes

- 1 large onion, sliced

- 1 red bell pepper, seeded and sliced

- 1/2 cup cashew, soaked overnight, crushed

- 1 tsp. dry mustard

- 2 tbsp. lemon juice

- 1/2 tsp. cayenne, oregano, cumin

- 1 tsp. salt, black pepper

- Extra virgin olive oil

- 4 flax tortillas

## Directions

1.  Peel sweet potato, chop and place in steamer for 20 minutes or until soft.

2.  Heat 2 tbsp. olive oil in skillet and sauté onion and bell pepper; add cashew and sauté for a minute, set aside.

3.  Mash sweet potato and mix with spices.

4.  Spoon a quarter of potato mixture into each wrap, top with sautéed onion, bell pepper and cashew, and roll into burrito.

**Nutrition**

Calories 345

Carbs 63

Fat 8

Protein 6

Sodium 21

**Avocado Shrimp Wrap**

Serves: 4

Prep Time: 10 mins.

## Ingredients

- 1 lb. shrimp, peeled, deveined

- 1 red bell pepper, seeded and chopped

- 1 medium onion, peeled, chopped

- 1/2 avocado, pitted

- 1 lemon, juiced

- 1/2 tsp. salt, black pepper

- 4 flax tortillas

## Directions

1. Mix shrimp with bell pepper and onion in glass bowl.

2. Place avocado in blender and mix until smooth, add lemon juice, salt, pepper.

3. Mix avocado into shrimp mixture and place a quarter of mixture into each flax tortilla.

# Chicken Lemon Cabbage Wraps

Serves: 4

Prep Time: 10 mins.

## Ingredients

- 1 lb. chicken breasts, roasted

- 1 red bell pepper, seeded, chopped

- 1 celery stalk, finely chopped

- 1 onion, peeled and chopped

- 4 cloves garlic

- 1 lemon, juiced

- 1/2 head cabbage

- 1 tsp. salt, pepper

## Directions

1.    Heat large pot of water until boiling.

2.    Separate cabbage leaves and place in boiling water for two minutes, remove and run under cold water.

3.    Chop chicken breasts into ½" pieces, place in large bowl and mix with remaining ingredients save cabbage.

4.  Spoon chicken mixture into cabbage leaves and secure roll with toothpick or enjoy open faced.

## Nutrition

- Calories 246

- Carbs 0

- Fat 10

- Protein 35

- Sodium 148

# Spinach Cheese Wrap

Serves: 4

Prep Time: 10 min.

## Ingredients

- 6 cups spinach, chopped

- 2 tomatoes, diced

- 1 small onion, minced

- 4 cloves garlic, minced

- 3/4 cup cashew, soaked overnight

- 1 tsp. salt, black pepper

- Extra virgin olive oil

- 4 cauliflower wraps

## Directions

1.   Place cashews in food processor with lemon juice and crush until crumbly.

2.   Heat olive oil in skillet; add onion, garlic and sauté for a minute.

3.   Add spinach, tomato and continue to sauté for two minutes.

4.   Reduce heat to low, add salt, pepper and cook for another five minutes.

5.   Spoon spinach into cauliflower wrap, sprinkle with cashew cheese and roll.

## Sausage and Pepper Wrap

Serves: 4

Prep Time: 10 mins.

## Ingredients

- 2 lean Italian sausage links

- 1 onion, sliced

- 2 red bell peppers

- 1 green bell pepper

- 4 cloves, garlic, minced

- Salt and pepper to taste

- Extra virgin olive oil

- 4 flax tortillas

## Directions

1. Slice sausage into ½" rounds.

2. Heat 2 tbsp. olive oil in skillet, add sausage, sauté.

3. Add bell peppers, onion, and garlic and continue to sauté until onion is golden brown.

4. Spoon sausage and peppers into flax tortilla.

## Nutrition

- Calories 180

- Carbs 14

- Fat 5

- Protein 20

- Sodium 640

## Tropical Mango Chicken

Serves: 4

Prep. Time: 10 mins.

### Ingredients

- 1 lb. chicken breasts

- 1/2 cup mango, chopped

- 1/4 cup parsley, chopped

- 2 tbsp. coconut cream

- 1 tsp. paprika

- 1 tsp. salt, black pepper

- Extra virgin olive oil

- 4 almond wraps

### Directions

1.  Combine mango, parsley, coconut cream in bowl, set aside.

2. Slice chicken breast into strips.

3. Heat 2 tbsp. olive oil in skillet; add chicken breast and sauté until golden brown.

4. Sprinkle with paprika, salt, pepper and spoon into wraps.

5. Top with mango chutney and roll them up.

## Nutrition

- Calories 321

- Carbs 19

- Fat 14

- Protein 35

- Sodium 148

## Apple Bacon Chicken Wrap

Serves: 4

Prep Time: 15 mins.

## Ingredients

- 4 slices bacon

- 3/4 lb. chicken breast, skinless, boneless

- 2 Granny Smith Apples, peeled, chopped

- 1 lemon, juiced

- 1/2 tsp. thyme

- 1 tsp. salt, black pepper

- Extra virgin olive oil

- 4 flax tortillas

## Directions

1. Coat 4 qt. slow cooker with olive oil.

2. Place apples in bottom of pot, top with chicken, bacon and spices.

3. Cook on low overnight for 8 hours.

## Nutrition

- Calories 318

- Carbs 23

- Fat 21

- Protein 35

- Sodium 843

# Tomato Zucchini Wrap

Serves: 4

Prep Time: 10 mins.

## Ingredients

- 2 tomatoes, chopped

- 1 cup basil, chopped

- 6 garlic cloves, minced

- 1 onion, chopped

- 4 zucchinis

- 1 tsp. oregano

- 1 tsp. salt, black pepper

## Directions

1. Preheat oven to 375 degrees and coat baking tray with olive oil.

2. Slice off ends of zucchini and using mandolin slice long strips, set aside.

3. Heat olive oil in skillet and sauté onion, garlic for a minute.

4.   In a bowl combine garlic mixture with tomato, basil, oregano, salt, black pepper.

5.   Place two strips zucchini on flat surface, spoon, tomato basil inside, roll up and secure with toothpick.

6.   Repeat with remaining ingredients and place in baking tray.

7.   Bake for 20 minutes.

## Nutrition

- Calories 117

- Carbs 12

- Fat 7

- Protein 3

- Sodium 22

# DINNER RECIPES

## Salmon, Cherry and Arugula Flax Seed Wrap

Serves: 2

Prep Time: 10 mins.

## Ingredients

- 6 oz. salmon, shredded

- 1 cup arugula

- 1 lemon, juiced

- 1/4 cup cherries, pitted, halved

- 1/4 tsp. salt

- 1/2 tsp. coarse black pepper

- 2 flaxseed tortillas

## Directions

1.    Toss together salmon, cherries, salt and pepper.

2.    Spoon half of salmon filling into each flax wrap, top with half cup of arugula and roll.

## Nutrition

- Calories 144

- Carbs 7

- Fat 5

- Protein 17

- Sodium 45

# Meatballs with Fresh Mint Sauce Wrap

Serves: 4

Prep Time: 20 mins.

## Ingredients

## Meatballs

- 1 lb. lean ground beef

- 5 cloves garlic, peeled, minced

- 2 tbsp. tomato puree

- 1 egg

- 1/2 tsp. cumin

- 1 tsp. each salt, pepper

## Mint Sauce

- 3 cups mint, stemmed, chopped

- 1 lemon, juiced

- 1/4 cup extra virgin olive oil

- 1/2 tsp. salt

- 1/2 tsp. cayenne

## Mediterranean Hummus Wrap

Serves: 4

Prep Time: 10 mins.

**Ingredients**

**Filling**

- 3 cups roasted turkey, shredded

- ¼ cup walnuts, crushed

- 1 tsp. paprika

- 1 lemon, juiced

- 1 tsp. salt, black pepper

**Paleo Hummus**

- 4 cups cauliflower florets

- 1 tbsp. organic tahini

- 4 cloves garlic, minced

- 2 tbsp. extra virgin olive oil

- 4 cauliflower wraps

## Directions

1. Place ingredients for Paleo Hummus in food processor and mix until semi-smooth.

2. Heat skillet and cook hummus for three minutes, set aside.

3. Mix turkey, walnuts, paprika, lemon, salt and pepper.

4. Spread hummus on cauliflower wraps, spoon filling on tortilla and wrap.

## Nutrition

- Calories 149

- Carbs 1

- Fat 6

- Protein 23

- Sodium 671

# Tex-Mex Wrap Explosion

Serves: 4

Prep Time: 10 mins

## Ingredients

- 1 lb. sirloin steak

- 4 cloves garlic, minced

- 2 onions, sliced

- 1 green bell pepper, seeded and sliced

- 1 lime, juiced

- 1 tsp. cayenne

- 1 tsp. each salt, pepper

- Extra virgin olive oil

- 4 flax wraps

## Directions

1. Slice sirloin steak into strips, set aside

2. Heat 2 tbsp. olive oil in skillet, add steak and stir-fry until browned.

3. Remove steak into bowl, set aside.

4. Add onion, bell pepper to skillet, sauté for two minutes.

5. Return steak into skillet, add spices, sauté for a minute.

6. Turn off heat, cover and allow to rest for 10 minutes.

7. Spoon ¼ of beef sauté into each wrap and drizzle with a little lime juice.

## Nutrition

- Calories 248

- Carbs 8

- Fat 7

- Protein 35

- Sodium 76

## Pomegranate Chicken in Lettuce Wraps

Serves: 4

Prep Time: 15 mins.

## Ingredients

- 1 lb. chicken breast

- 1/2 cup pomegranate seeds

- 1 lemon juiced

- 1/4 cup walnuts, chopped

- 8 large Romaine lettuce leaves

- Extra virgin olive oil

## Directions

1. Slice chicken breast into thin strips.

2. Place 2 tbsp. olive oil in skillet and sauté chicken until golden brown.

3. Add nuts and pomegranate seeds, sauté for two minutes.

4. Squeeze lemon juice on top, cover and allow to cool.

5. lay down two pieces romaine lettuce and spoon chicken pomegranate chicken into leaves and roll into wrap.

## Nutrition

- Calories 347

- Carbs 14

- Fat 23

- Protein 39

- Sodium 145

# Paleo Pesto Chicken Wrap

Serves: 4

Prep Time: 15 mins.

## Ingredients

- 1 lb. chicken breasts, boneless, skinless

- 1 onion, diced

- 8 cloves garlic,

- 1 cup fresh basil

- ¼ cup pine nuts

- ½ cup cashews, soaked overnight

- ½ cup water

- 1 tsp. salt, pepper

- Extra virgin olive oil

- 4 cauliflower wraps

## Directions

1.  Preheat oven to 375 degrees and coat baking dish with olive oil.

2.     Place basil, garlic, pine nuts, cashews, salt, pepper, water and ¼ cup olive oil in food processor and mix until smooth, set aside.

3.     Place chicken in baking dish and coat with ¾ of basil mixture, bake in oven for 30 minutes turning halfway.

4.     Slice chicken into strips, place on wraps and spoon a little remaining basil mixture in each wrap.

## Nutrition

- Calories 393

- Carbs 11

- Fat 22

- Protein 37

- Sodium 102

# Stuffed Italian Wrap

Serves: 4

Prep Time: 10 mins.

## Ingredients

- 1 lb. lean ground beef

- 2 cups tomato puree

- 4 cups cauliflower florets

- 1 onion, diced

- 4 cloves garlic, minced

- 1 tsp. oregano

- 4 cloves, ground

- 1 basil leaf

- 1 tsp. salt, black pepper

- Extra virgin olive oil

- 4 almond wraps

**Directions**

1.  Place cauliflower florets in food processor and puree until rice-like granules form.

2.  Heat 2 tbsp. olive oil in skillet; add onion, garlic and sauté for a minute.

3.  Add beef and brown.

4.  Add tomato, cloves, salt, and pepper, turn heat to low and simmer for 10 minutes.

5.  Add cauliflower, simmer for another five minutes.

6.   Remove basil leaf, spoon mixture into wraps and roll tightly.

**Nutrition**

- Calories 299

- Carbs 20

- Fat 7

- Protein 39

- Sodium 140

# Pork and Sweet Potato Comfort Wrap

Serves: 4

Prep Time: 10 mins.

**Ingredients**

- 1 lb. pork chops, boneless

- 1 sweet potato, peeled and cubed

- 1 onion, diced

- 1 tsp. fresh rosemary

- 1 tsp. salt, black pepper

- Extra virgin olive oil

- 4 almond wraps

## Directions

1. Steam sweet potato for 20 minutes.

2. Slice pork chops into strips.

3. In skillet, heat 2 tbsp. olive oil, sauté onion and garlic for a minute, add pork strips, and continue to sauté for another five minutes.

4. Cover, reduce heat and allow to sit for 10 minutes.

5. Mash sweet potato with ghee, rosemary, salt, pepper.

6. Spoon sweet potato into wrap and top with pork strips.

## Nutrition

- Calories 466

- Carbs 24

- Fat 28

- Protein 28

- Sodium 116

## Creamy Salty Crab Wraps

Serves: 4

Prep Time: 10 mins.

**Ingredients**

- 2 cups crab meat

- 1 celery stalk, chopped

- 1/2 cup cashews, soaked overnight

- 2 tbsp. coconut cream

- 1/2 tsp. dry mustard

- 1 lemon, juiced

- 1 tsp. cayenne

- 1 tsp. each salt and pepper

- Extra virgin olive oil

- 4 cauliflower wraps

## Directions

1. Place cashews in food processor and mix until crumbly, add coconut cream and mix until smooth, add a little water if required.

2. Mix cashew with crab meat, celery and spices.

3. Spoon into cauliflower wraps.

## Nutrition

- Calories 129

- Carbs 6

- Fat 10

- Protein 5

- Sodium 95

## Swedish Shrimp Salad Wrap

Serves: 4

Prep Time: 10 mins.

## Ingredients

- 1 lb. medium shrimp, peeled, deveined

- 1/4 cup dill, chopped

- 1 small red onion, chopped

- 2 tbsp. coconut cream

- 1 tsp. salt, pepper

- 1 egg, hard-boiled

- 4 flax tortillas

## Directions

1. Place dill, coconut cream, salt, pepper and egg in blender and mix until creamy.

2. Mix dill sauce with shrimp, red onion and wrap in flax tortillas.

**Nutrition**

- Calories 140

- Carbs 4

- Fat 3

- Protein 25

- Sodium 264

# CONCLUSION

Thanks again for downloading my book, as you can see, Paleo diet can help stabilize the blood sugar level of a person. This is the reason why diabetics are recommended to try this diet. This kind of diet can also improve energy level that enables an individual to accomplish more tasks the whole day. Consuming Paleo breakfast recipes also boosts the efficiency of workout routines. There are other benefits that individuals will experience in this diet like stronger teeth, better complexion, and enhanced sleeping patterns.

Paleo diet recipes are popular as they have helped lots of folks in steering clear from heart ailments. Furthermore, this diet enhances the immune system. Meaning to say, individuals who choose cooking their own Paleo dessert recipes can steer clear of diseases like common colds and flu.

Because of the many health advantages that it brings, it's no longer surprising why paleo diet became one of the most searched subjects in the internet.

In order for stuff to fall into place, you need to use **paleo diet** by utilizing all the information that we have in this book. Quick and fast approach is not a bad thing, however, you also have to patiently wait and commit to a long term plan for your healthy life.

Please take some time to leave a review of my book on Amazon and also don't forget to check out my other books here.

MARIA COOK

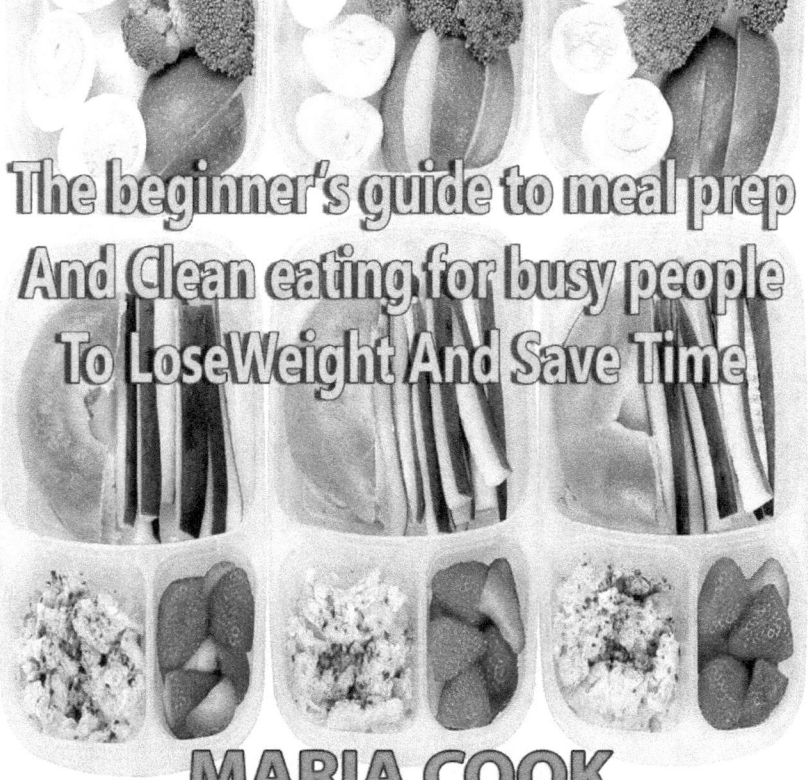

# MEAL PREP

The beginner's guide to meal prep
And Clean eating for busy people
To LoseWeight And Save Time

## MARIA COOK

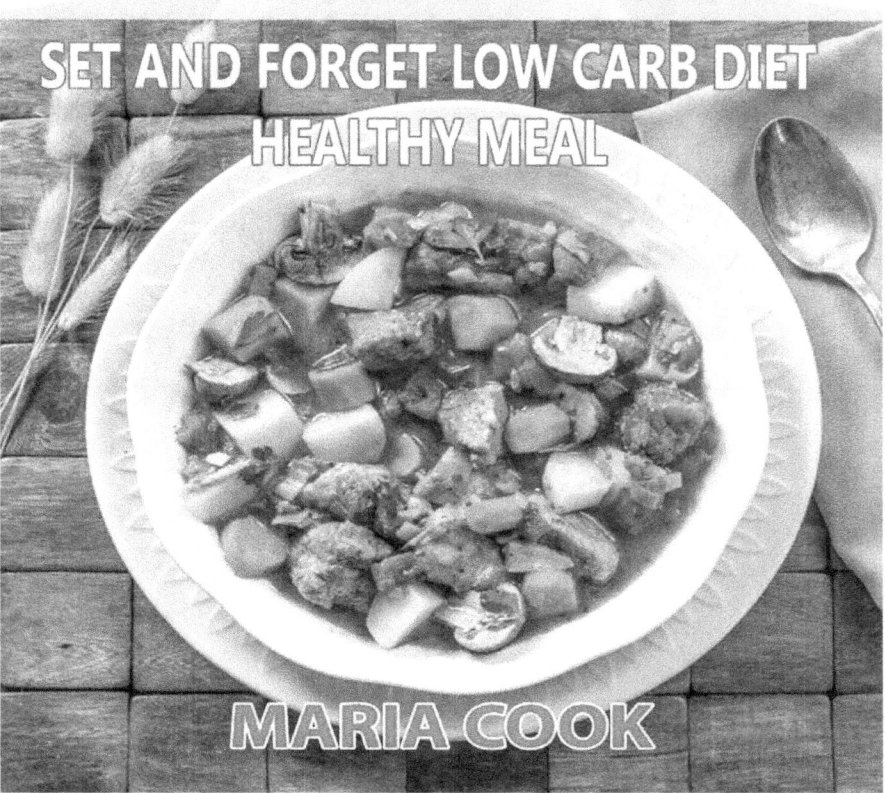

Slow Cooker Cookbook

# SLOW COOKER

*The Guide to "Set and Forget" Cooking*

*Style Using Your Ultimate*

**Slow Cooker**

**Maria Cook**

# SLOW COOKER COOKBOOK

A Slow Cooker (SLOW COOKER) is essential in the kitchen of any busy family. When time is limited most people end up in the fast food drive thru somewhere ordering food that is very unhealthy habit and also leaving a hole in your pocket too.

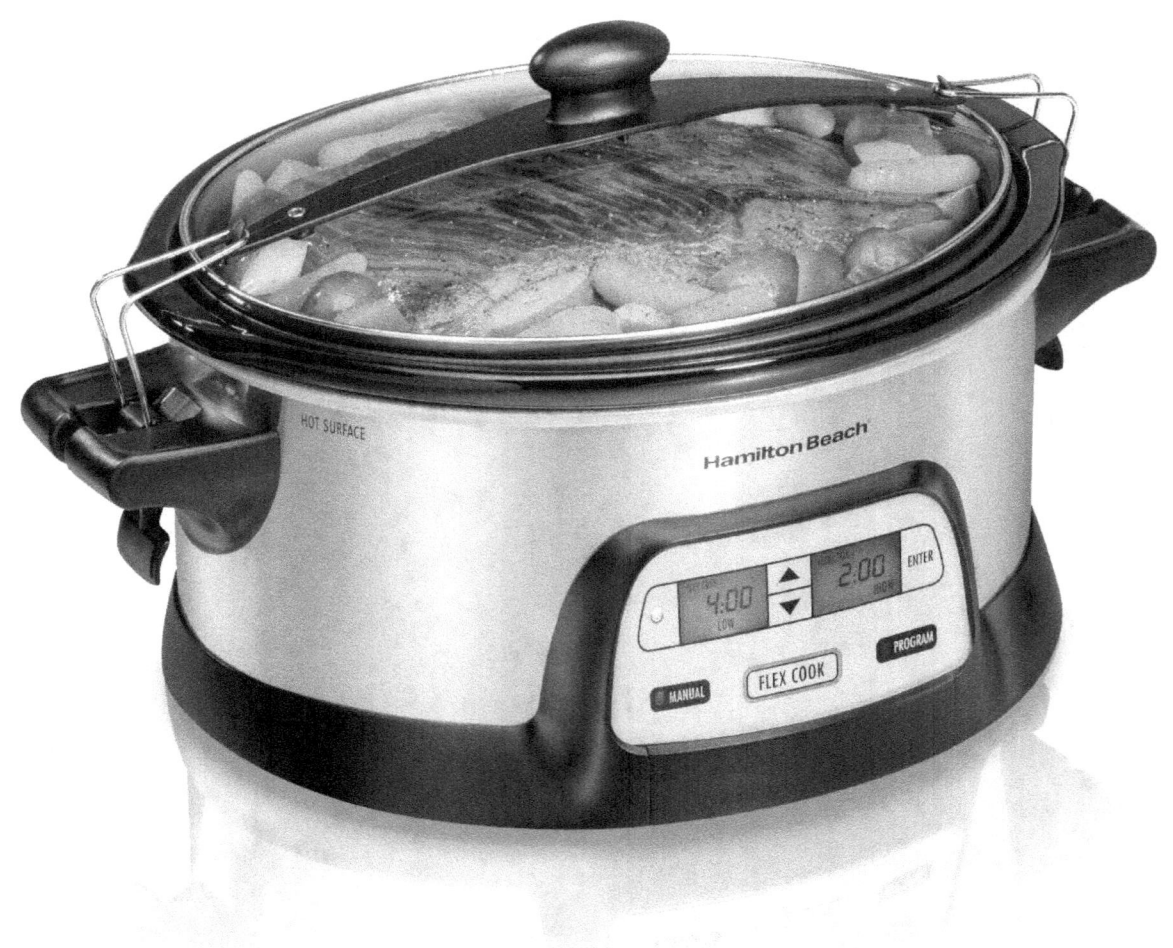

Getting a Slow Cooker will put an end to the unhealthy meals on days when you just don't have time to stop and cook a nice meal. You can throw in whatever foods you have readily on hand and let it cook while you while you are off working, going to school, or playing carpool with the kids, saving heap of time for yourself.

Here are just some basic ways to use one of these cookers.

Soup: you can make your own soups with literally whatever is on hand, and it will taste delicious. Just put some chicken broth in the crockpot and add in fresh or frozen vegetables and some sort of meat if you want. Chicken cut into small chunks works well. Fill up close to the top with water and let the meat cook overnight or all day.

The best benefit of using the slow cooker for cooking is that the dishes you are preparing stay nutritious. Using mainly fresh and healthy ingredients for your slow cooker meals, the ingredients will be cooked at a low temperature for a long time, therefore they become extremely tender and delicious. Since there is only a little evaporation the food will never dry out. The natural juices of the meat and vegetables are kept in the pot, so the food is both nutritious and juicy. Therefore, if you are looking for healthy food, using the slow cooker to prepare meals is the way to reach a perfect result.

Slow cooker can cook stews and soups but they are great for cooking inexpensive, tough cuts of meat. By cooking sides or desserts in the slow cooker, you are creating another burner or oven. When entertaining, your oven usually gets occupied by large, long-cooking dishes.

If you spray the slow cooker with nonstick spray before you begin cooking, it will make cleanup easier.

Meats don't brown in a crock pot. If a recipe calls for the meat to be browned, you will need to brown the meat before adding it to the crock pot.

Cooking in a slow cooker retains moisture so even though you might be tempted, you don't need to add any more liquid than the recipe calls for.

Cooking times will vary as with any appliance. There are many factors that will affect cooking times. The amount of food in the pot. The humidity. How hot the foods are that you put in the crock pot. Cooking times in recipes are just ranges.

You can also transform almost all your traditional recipes for the slow cooker; just reduce the liquid by at least 50 percent because there is virtually no loss of steam during the cooking since it is covered, therefore sauces do not reduce much which increase the cooking time. In average one hour in the oven is equivalent of about 6 to 8 hours on low (divide by two for high which will comprise 3 to 4 hours) in your slow cooker.

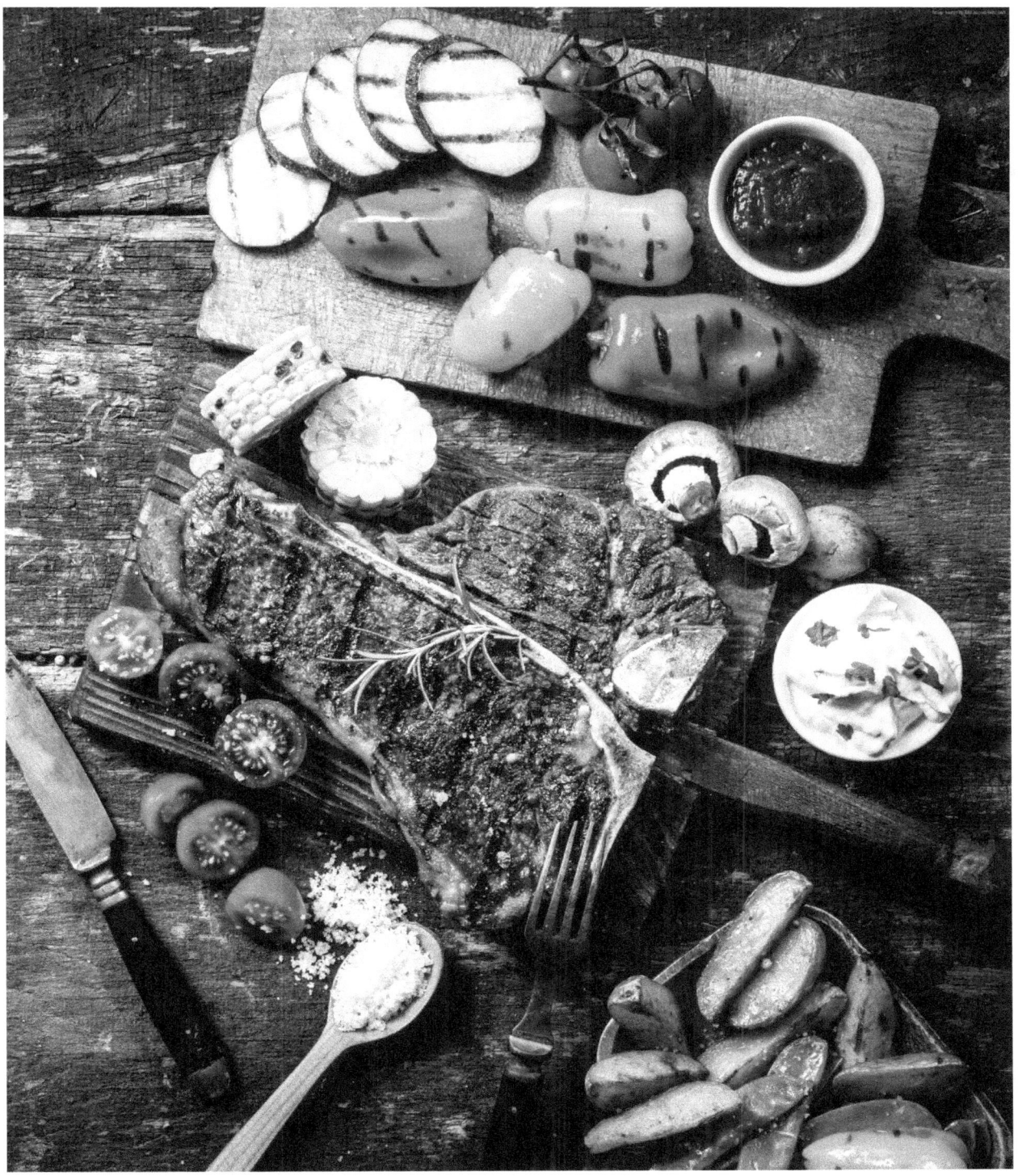

As its name suggests, the slow cooker is designed to cook food slowly with indirect heat. Existed already for around 30 years the low cookers were forgotten for a while and it is just great that they came back to our routine life during recent years with more comfortable design and better performance.

It will allow you to save money as well since you will be using 80% less energy than while cooking on a traditional stove.

You can make some healthy substitutions that will not distract from the taste. In fact, some of the alternative ingredients that are beloved by many chefs will enhance the flavor and add to it.

For instance, substituting some of the common ingredients can easily make a meal healthier all around.

Here are a few alternatives you can choose from:

- All-purpose white flour = white wheat (can be bought from any store)

- White sugar = honey granules or coconut sugar

- Cornstarch = arrowroot

- Canola or vegetable oil = olive oil or coconut oil

- Whole milk = coconut milk

When you bake a dessert in your slow cooker, you'll need to have the right tools. These will include parchment paper, ramekins, baking dishes that are round and will fit in your cooker, mitts, and baking inserts.

# SLOW COOKER TIPS

TIP # 1. Remove the lid when the time is done by lifting it so that the steam goes away from you and not directly up in your face. You won't want to keep lifting the lid while it's cooking because letting out the heat will prolong the cooking time and cause your food to cook incorrectly. Avoid this by following the instructions and leaving it alone. If you're cooking overnight or throughout the day while you're gone, you won't have that temptation. Whatever you do, avoid lifting that lid!

TIP # 2. You can use your slow cooker to make delicious caramel. Instead of letting it burn trying to cook it on your stovetop, put it in your slow cooker so you can control it better. In fact, the recipe for making caramel in a slow cooker is so simple and easy, anyone at all can do it. Just take two cans of condensed milk, leave them sealed and put them in your crockpot. Cover them completely with water and turn on your slow cooker. Heat them on low for 8 or 10 hours. Do not let them be out of the water at any time. If the water goes down, refill it. This is one recipe that allows you to lift the lid to check whenever you feel you need to.

Try to follow the recipes in the next part of this book as closely as you can to get the very result. If you need to make some adjustments, feel free to do so. Especially once you've mastered your cooker you can use your slow cooker combined with you cooking skills to make the best creative meals and the numbers of recipes will be unlimited.

# SLOW COOKER BREAKFAST RECIPES

Preparing great breakfasts is often a challenge for large families and those who find it difficult to get up early in the morning and prepare something great.

Besides the challenge of having to constantly think of easy ways to prepare great morning meals.

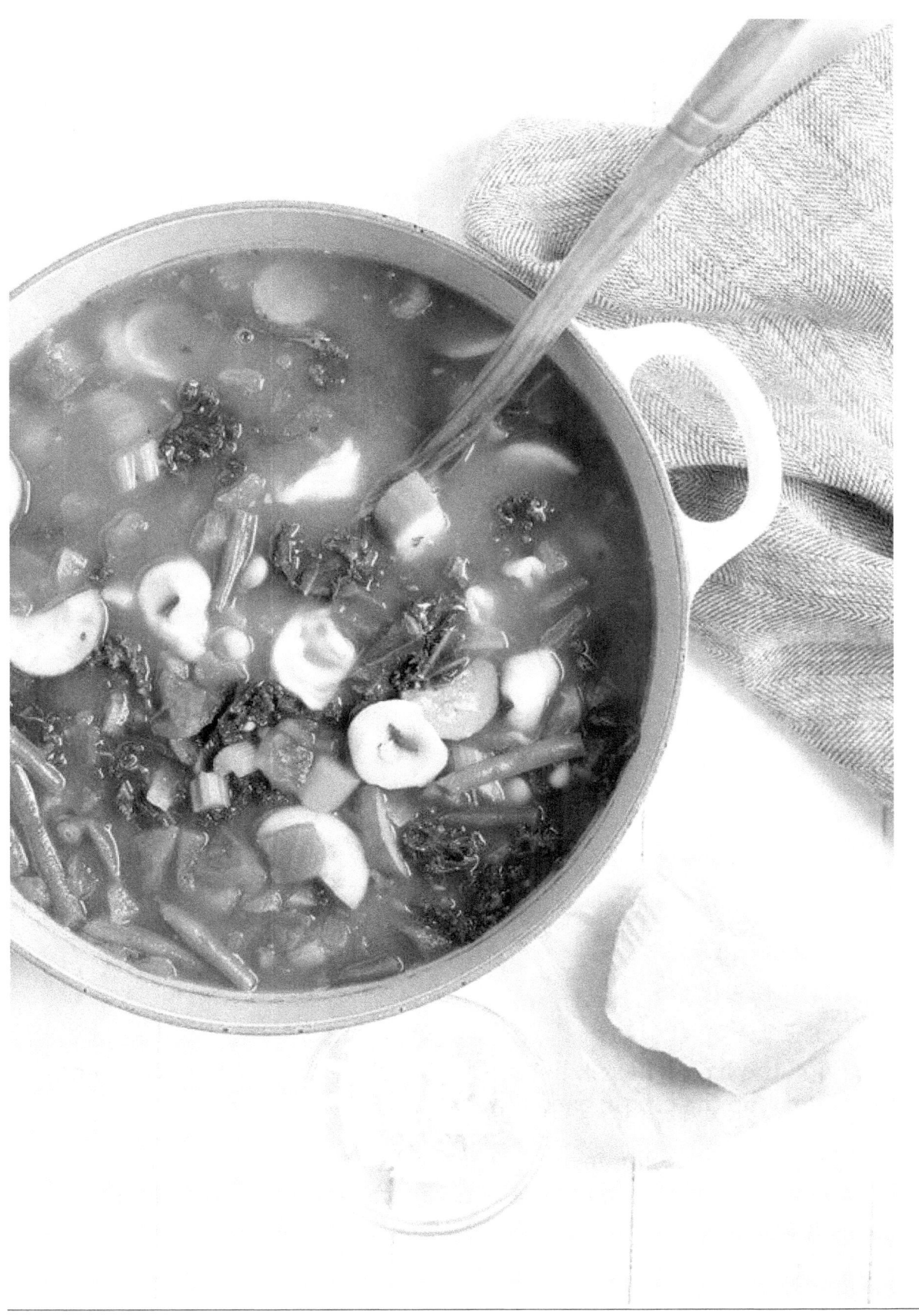

# BREAKFAST DELIGHT CASSEROLE

- Yield: 8

- Time taken: 10 hours

**Ingredients:**

- ✓ 1 onion (peeled and chopped)

- ✓ 8 strips of bacon

- ✓ 1 red bell pepper (seeded and chopped)

- ✓ 1 cup broccoli (chopped)

- ✓ 1 clove of garlic (minced)

- ✓ 1 cup mushroom (chopped)

- ✓ 1 cup milk (with 2% fat)

- ✓ 12 eggs

- ✓ 1½ cheddar cheese (shredded)

- ✓ 2 bags of hash browns

- ✓ ½ tsp salt

- ✓ ½ tsp pepper

- ✓ 1 tsp dried dill

**Directions:**

1. Cook the bacon in a skillet until crisp. Spread it on a plate to cool and then chop the crispy bacon in strips.

2. Chop onions, bell pepper, garlic, broccoli and mushrooms and sauté them in the skillet using the leftover bacon grease for 5 minutes until slightly tender.

3. Coat the slow cooker with cooking spray and place one-third of the hash browns at the bottom of the cooker and season with salt and pepper.

4. Lay one-third portion of the sautéed vegetables along with one-third portion of cheese.

5. Repeat this order of layering till all the ingredients are used. The top layer should be cheese.

6. In a large bowl, blend eggs with milk, dill, salt and pepper and pour the liquid over the top of the layers in the cooker.

7. Place a paper towel under the lid of the cooker so that excess moisture can be absorbed while cooking and then cover the cooker.

8. Cook on low setting for 8 to 10 hours.

9. Serve hot.

## *DELIGHTFUL COFFEE CAKE*

- Yield: 8

- Time taken: 2 hours 10 minutes

**Ingredients:**

**For streusel topping:**

- ✓ ¼ cup packed light brown sugar

- ✓ ¼ cup biscuit baking mix

- ✓ ½ tsp cinnamon

**For batter:**

- ✓ ¾ cup white sugar

- ✓ 1½ cup biscuit baking mix

- ✓ ½ cup vanilla yogurt

- ✓ 1 tsp vanilla

- ✓ 1 large egg

**For glazed icing:**

- ✓ 2 tbsps. Milk

- ✓ ½ cup sugar

**Directions:**

1. Grease the crockpot with cooking spray and place a piece of parchment paper to fit the bottom of the pot and coat the paper with cooking spray as well.

2. Put all the streusel topping ingredients in a bowl and blend them well. Keep the bowl aside.

3. Put all the batter ingredients in another bowl and heat to make a smooth batter.

4. Pour half portion of the batter into the pot using a spoon and sprinkle half of the streusel mixture over the batter. Repeat the layering with the remaining ingredients.

5. Line the lid with a paper towel and cook the cake on high for 2 hours. Check with a toothpick to see if the cake is ready. Cook for a few more minutes if required.

6. While the cake cooks make the glazed icing by mixing the milk with powdered sugar and keep aside.

7. Once the cake is ready, invert the pot on a serving plate and top it with the glazed icing.

8. Cut into slices and serve.

## *HOMEMADE CARAMEL ROLLS*

- Yield: 8

- Time taken: 1 hour 15 minutes

**Ingredients:**

- ✓ 4 tbsps. Butter

- ✓ ½ cup brown sugar

- ✓ 1 packet of cinnamon rolls

**Directions:**

1. Spray the slow cooker with cooking spray and keep aside.

2. Melt butter in a saucepan and add brown sugar to make a thick paste. Cook for 3 minutes to make the caramel sauce.

3. Put the cinnamon rolls into the slow cooker and pour the caramel sauce over the rolls.

4. Cook on high setting for 1 hour and serve.

# *POTATO CASSEROLE DELIGHT*

- Yield: 8

- Time taken: 8 hours 10 minutes

**Ingredients:**

- ✓ 1 lb. bacon

- ✓ 1 bag of frozen hash brown potatoes

- ✓ ½ red bell pepper

- ✓ 1 small onion (diced)

- ✓ 8 oz. shredded cheddar cheese

- ✓ 12 eggs

- ✓ 1 cup milk

- ✓ ½ green bell pepper

- ✓ Salt and pepper

**Directions:**

1. Cut the bacon in small pieces and cook until crisp.

2. Coat the crockpot with cooking spray and layer it with half portion of hash browns at the bottom followed by half portions of onion, bacon, red and green peppers and cheese. Repeat the layering and make sure that the top layer is made with cheese.

3. Beat the eggs and add milk with it and remember to season with salt and pepper.

4. Pour the egg mixture over the layers in the pot and cook for 8 hours on low setting.

# *PUMPKIN BREAD PUDDING*

- • Yield: 6 cups

- • Time taken: 1 hour 40 minutes

**Ingredients:**

- ✓ 3 eggs (beaten)

- ✓ 2 cups of skimmed milk

- ✓ 1½ cups pure pumpkin puree

- ✓ 1 tsp cinnamon

- ✓ ¼ cup brown sugar

- ✓ ½ tsp nutmeg

- ✓ ¼ tsp cloves

- ✓ ¾ tsp orange zest

- ✓ ½ tsp ginger

- ✓ 8 cup white bread cubes

- ✓ 1½ cup wheat bran

- ✓ Caramel sauce

**Directions:**

1. Blend the pumpkin puree with milk, beaten eggs, cinnamon, brown sugar, nutmeg, orange zest, cloves and ginger in a bowl and keep aside.

2. Coat the slow cooker with cooking spray and keep ready.

3. Now put the bread cubes in the pumpkin mixture and pour the entire mixture into the slow cooker.

4. Cook on high setting for 1 hour 30 minutes and serve warm.

## *GRANOLA WITH SALTED ALMONDS*

- • Yield: 6 cups

- • Time taken: 2 hours 10 minutes

**Ingredients:**

- ✓ 1 cup salted caramel almonds

- ✓ 5 cups rolled oats

- ✓ ¼ cup almond butter

- ✓ ½ cup melted coconut oil

- ✓ 1 tsp vanilla extract

- ✓ ½ cup honey

✓ ½ tsp caramel extract

✓ 1½ tsp salt

**Directions:**

1. Coat a large crockpot with cooking spray and add almonds and oats in it. Toss them to mix properly.

2. Mix butter with oil, vanilla extract, honey, salt and caramel extract in a small bowl. Warm this mixture up for 30 seconds in a microwave.

3. Pour this mixture over the mixture of almonds and oats and toss well to combine.

4. Cover the cooker and cook on high setting for 2 hours.

5. Garnish with chocolate chips and serve in bowls.

## *BUTTER PANCAKE IN A SLOW COOKER*

- Yield: 6

- Time taken: 1 hour 5 minutes

**Ingredients:**

✓ 1 cup milk

✓ 6 eggs

✓ 1 cup flour

✓ ½ tsp salt

✓ 4 tbsps. Melted butter

**Directions:**

1. Mix milk with flour, eggs and salt in a bowl.

2. Coat the slow cooker with cooking spray and melt the butter in it.

3. Pour the batter in it and cook by covering the cooker for 1 hour on high setting.

4. The pancake cooks until it is puffed up.

5. Serve with a syrup of your choice.

# *BLUEBERRY BISCUIT WITH LEMON ICING*

- Yield: 6

- Time taken: 5 hours 10 minutes

**Ingredients:**

**For the cake:**

- ✓ 1 cup frozen blueberries

- ✓ 7.5 oz. prepared biscuit dough

- ✓ ¼ cup sugar

- ✓ 1 tbsp. melted butter

- ✓ 1 tsp cornstarch

**For lemon icing:**

- ✓ 1 cup powdered sugar

- ✓ 2 tbsps. Lemon juice

- ✓ 3 tbsps. Milk

**Directions:**

1. Coat the SLOW COOKER using non-stick cooking spray.

2. Toss the blueberries with sugar and cornstarch in a bowl and cut each biscuit into quarters.

3. Put half portion of biscuit in the pot and sprinkle the blueberry mixture and then repeat the layering with the remaining portion of ingredients.

4. Brush the top layer with melted butter and cook on low for 5 hours.

5. While the cake is cooking, make the icing by mixing all the ingredients.

6. When the cake is ready and out of the pot, drizzle it with the icing mixture and serve by slicing into pieces.

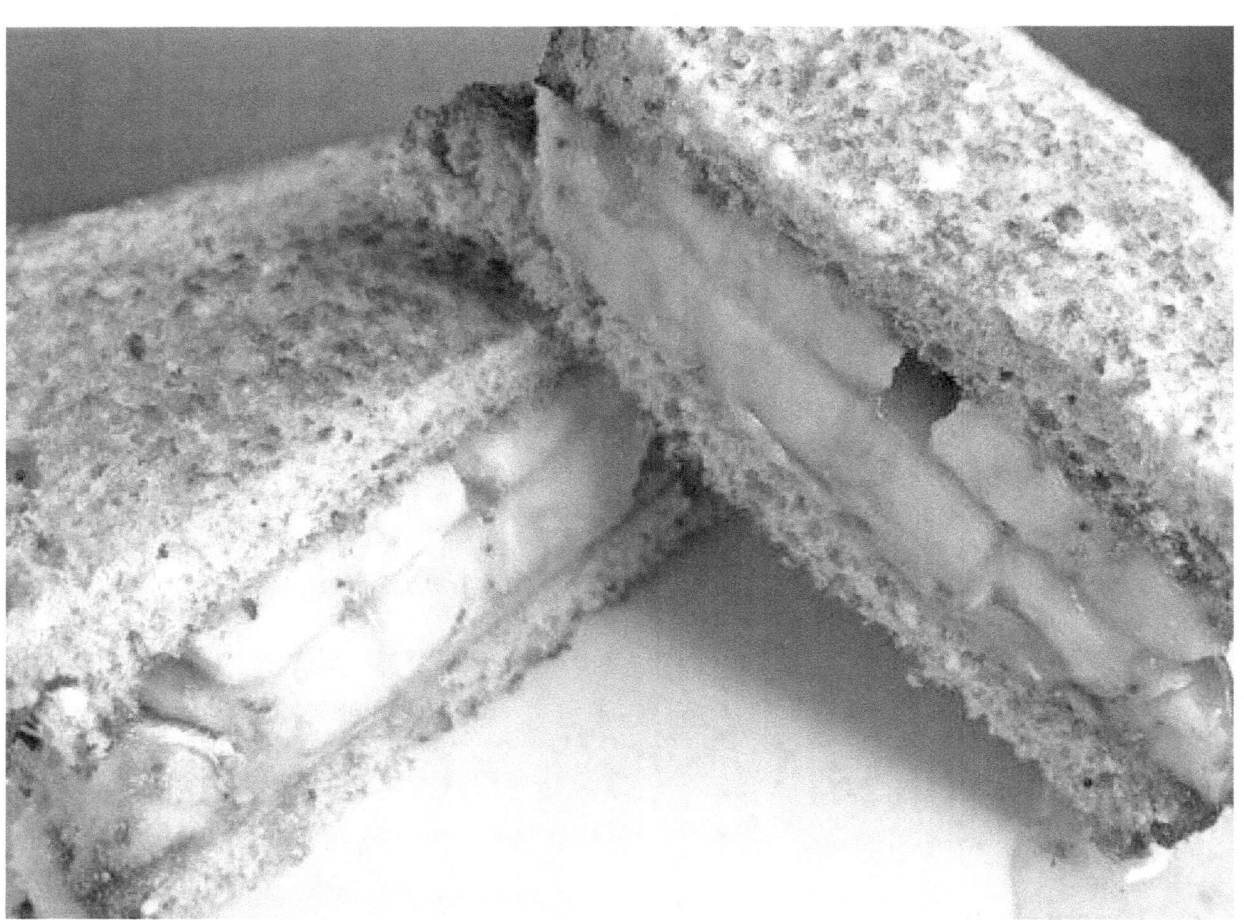

## POTATO AND SAUSAGE CASSEROLE

- Yield: 6

- Time taken: 6 hours 5 minutes

**Ingredients:**

- ✓ 6 eggs
- ✓ ½ lb. ground sausage
- ✓ Salt and pepper
- ✓ ½ cup milk
- ✓ ½ cup salsa
- ✓ 1 lb. frozen hash browns
- ✓ 1 cup cheddar cheese (shredded)

**Directions:**

1. Coat the slow cooker with non-stick cooking spray.

2. Beat the eggs in a bowl and then add the milk along with pepper and salt.

3. Pour the mixture into the cooker and add the sausage along with hash browns, cheese and salsa.

4. Cover the pot and cook on low setting for 6 hours, making sure that the eggs and potatoes are cooked properly.

## *TATER TOTS WITH BACON & EGGS*

- Yield: 8
- Time taken: 8 hours 15 minutes

**Ingredients:**

- ✓ 6 oz. bacon
- ✓ 1 packet of Tater Tots
- ✓ 2 cup cheddar cheese (shredded)
- ✓ 2 onions (chopped)

- ✓ 12 eggs

- ✓ ¼ cup grated parmesan cheese

- ✓ 1 tsp salt

- ✓ 1 cup milk

- ✓ ½ tsp pepper

- ✓ 4 tbsps. All-purpose flour

**Directions:**

1. Coat the crockpot with cooking spray and layer the bottom with one-third portion of tater tots followed by one-third portion of bacon, onion and cheese.

2. Repeat the layering with the remaining portions of ingredients ensuring the top layer is made with cheese.

3. Whisk the eggs with the remaining ingredients in a bowl and pour it on top.

4. Cover the cooker and cook on low setting for 8 hours.

## HAM & EGG SPINACH BREAKFAST

- Yield: 6

- Time taken: 2 hours 5 minutes

**Ingredients:**

- ✓ ¼ cup milk

- ✓ 6 large eggs

- ✓ ½ tsp salt

- ✓ ¼ tsp black pepper

- ✓ ½ cup Greek yogurt
- ✓ ½ tsp onion powder
- ✓ ½ tsp thyme
- ✓ ½ tsp garlic powder
- ✓ 1 cup baby spinach
- ✓ 1/3 cup diced mushrooms
- ✓ 1 cup pepper jack cheese
- ✓ 1 cup diced ham

**Directions:**

1. Whisk the eggs, pepper, salt, yogurt, milk, thyme, garlic powder and onion powder in a bowl to make a smooth paste.

2. Add the spinach and mushrooms along with cheese and ham.

3. Coat the cooker with cooking spray and pour the mixture into it.

4. Cover and cook for 2 hours and serve after slicing into pieces.

# *CHEESY SAUSAGE CASSEROLE*

- Yield: 8

- Time taken: 4 hours 15 minutes

**Ingredients:**

- ✓ 1 lb. ground sausage
- ✓ 32 oz. frozen hash brown
- ✓ 1½ cheddar cheese (grated)
- ✓ ½ cup milk

- ✓ 1 cup Mozzarella cheese

- ✓ 1½ cup jack cheese (grated)

- ✓ 1 tbsp. Creole seasoning

- ✓ ½ cup sliced green onion

- ✓ ½ tbsp. black pepper

- ✓ ½ tbsp. onion powder

- ✓ ½ tbsp. garlic powder

- ✓ Olive oil

- ✓ 12 eggs (beaten)

**Directions:**

1. Mix the seasoning blend and keep aside.

2. Heat one tablespoon of olive oil in a pan and cook the sausage with the seasoning blend for 10 minutes until the sausage is brown in color.

3. Spray the cooker with cooking spray and then make a layer of ½ portions of potatoes and sprinkle the seasoning mixture.

4. Now make a layer of half portion of cooked sausage and top with cheese layer. Repeat the layering with the remaining ingredients and make the top layer with cheese.

5. Blend the eggs with milk and remaining seasoning and pour over the top.

6. Cook for 4 hours on high setting and serve by garnishing with green onions.

# APPLE HONEY GRANOLA

- Yield: 2

- Time taken: 8 hrs. 10 minutes

**Ingredients:**

- ✓ 2 cups of gluten-free granola
- ✓ 4 apples (peeled and sliced)
- ✓ 1 tsp cinnamon
- ✓ 2 tbsps. Melted coconut oil
- ✓ ¼ cup honey

**Directions:**

1. Grease the SLOW COOKER with cooking spray and place the apple slices in it.

2. Mix the remaining ingredients in a bowl and top the with the apple slices.

3. Cover the cooker and cook on low setting for 8 hours.

# *FRUITY AND SPICY OATS*

- Yield: 2
- Time taken: 8 hours 5 minutes

**Ingredients:**

- ✓ 1 tbsp. melted butter
- ✓ 2 cups of milk
- ✓ ¼ cup brown sugar
- ✓ 1 cup rolled oats
- ✓ ½ tsp cinnamon

✓ ¼ tsp salt

✓ ½ cup raisins

✓ ½ cup walnuts (crushed)

✓ 1 cup chopped apples

**Directions:**

1. Coat the cooker with cooking spray and then put all the ingredients in it and mix using a spatula until the ingredients are evenly mixed.

2. Cover the slow cooker and cook on low setting for 8 hours.

## *CARAMELED NUT BISCUITS*

- Yield: 8 biscuits

- Time taken: 2 hours

**Ingredients:**

✓ ½ cup brown sugar

✓ 8 pieces Frozen biscuits (any flavor of your choice)

✓ 4 tbsps. Butter

✓ Nuts for garnishing

**Directions:**

1. Coat the crockpot with cooking spray and lay the biscuits flat at the bottom.

2. Use a saucepan to melt the butter and mix the brown sugar and cook for a few minutes to caramelize it.

3. Pour half portion of the caramelized sugar over the biscuits and cook in the crockpot for 1 hour 30 minutes.

4. Now preheat the oven at 350 degrees and spray non-stick cooking spray in the baking dish.

5. Place the cooked biscuits on the tray and pour the remaining caramel mixture on them.

6. Cook for 20 minutes and serve.


# CASSEROLE WITH SMOKED CHEESE

- Yield: 8

- Time taken: 5 hours 40 minutes

**Ingredients:**

- ✓ 2 tbsps. Butter

- ✓ 10 cups of cubed French bread

- ✓ 9 eggs

- ✓ 8 oz. sliced fresh mushrooms

- ✓ ½ tsp red pepper flakes

- ✓ 2 cups "half-n-half"

- ✓ 1 lb. bacon (thick slices)

- ✓ 1 green bell pepper (coarsely chopped)

- ✓ ¼ cup chopped parsley

- ✓ 2 cups smoked cheddar cheese (shredded)

**Directions:**

1. Keep the oven ready by preheating at 300 degrees.

2. Spread the bread cubes on a cookie sheet and bake them for 30 minutes until they become dry.

3. Melt butter in a skillet and cook the mushrooms in it for 5 minutes.

4. Beat the eggs and add the pepper flakes with half-n-half.

5. Put ¾ cup of cheese aside and mix the remaining with the egg mixture and then stir in the bacon, 2 tablespoons of parsley and bell pepper into it.

6. Now, fold in the bread cubes and stir well to coat.

7. Pour the mixture into the crockpot and cook by covering it on low setting for 5 hours.

8. Now, remove the cover and sprinkle the remaining parsley and reserved cheese on top and cook for another 10 minutes so that the cheese can melt.

# *FRUITY NUTTY CASSEROLE*

- Yield: 8

- Time taken: 5 hours 50 minutes

**Ingredients:**

**For casserole:**

- ✓ 1 loaf of French bread (cut into 1 inch cubes)

- ✓ ¼ cup granulated sugar

- ✓ 2 cups half-n-half (mixture of light cream and whole milk)

- ✓ 2 tbsps. Butter

- ✓ 3 eggs

- ✓ 1 tbsp. vanilla

- ✓ ¼ cup packed brown sugar

- ✓ 1 cup pecans (coarsely chopped)

- ✓ 1/8 tsp ground nutmeg

- ✓ ½ tsp ground cinnamon

**For caramel-banana sauce:**

- ✓ ½ cup whipping cream

- ✓ ½ cup butter

- ✓ 1 tsp vanilla

- ✓ 1 banana (thinly sliced)

- ✓ 2 tbsps. Light colored corn syrup

- ✓ ¾ cup packed brown sugar

**Directions:**

1. Make the caramel banana sauce by mixing the brown sugar with cream, butter and corn syrup and heat them in a pan. Bring the mixture to boil while whisking occasionally and then reduce the heat. Cook for 3 minutes by covering the pan.

2. Pour in another pan, cover it and place it in the fridge to chill.

3. Make the crockpot ready by lining it with a disposable cooker liner and keep the oven ready by preheating at 300 degrees.

4. Place the bread cubes on a baking sheet and bake for 15 minutes making sure that they are golden in color.

5. Then place the bread cubes in crockpot.

6. Whisk the eggs with half-n-half, granulated sugar, cinnamon, nutmeg, and vanilla in a bowl and pour the mixture over the bread cubes in the pot.

7. Use a pastry blender to cut the butter and blend with brown sugar till the butter is chopped into the size of peas and mix with the pecans. Sprinkle this mixture over the bread mixture in the pot.

8. Cover the pot and cook on low setting for 5 hours.

9. Remove the casserole from the pot and serve by topping with the caramel banana sauce and some fresh slices of banana.

# DELIGHTFUL HAM IN CROCKPOT

- Yield: 8

- Time taken: 4 hours 20 minutes:

**Ingredients:**

- ✓ 2/3 cup of half-n-half

- ✓ 12 eggs

- ✓ ½ tsp freshly ground black pepper

- ✓ ½ tsp salt

- ✓ ½ cup green onions (chopped)

- ✓ ½ tsp ground red pepper

- ✓ 4 oz. cheddar cheese (shredded)

- ✓ 1 cup Gruyere cheese (shredded)

- ✓ 9 oz. frozen spinach (thawed and drained)

- ✓ 6 cups country style hash browns (shredded)

- ✓ 2 cups of cooked ham (cubed)

**Directions:**

1. Prepare the crockpot by lining it with a foil and coating it with cooking spray.

2. Beat the eggs with salt, black pepper, half-n-half and red pepper in a bowl.

3. Keep aside ¾ cup of cheddar cheese and 2 tablespoons of green onions and mix them together in a separate bowl.

4. Layer half portion of potatoes at the bottom of the lined SLOW COOKER followed by spinach, ham, green onions and cheese. Repeat the layering order and make the top layer with cheese.

5. Pour the egg mixture on top and cover the pot.

6. Cook on low setting for 4 hours ensuring the egg is properly set.

7. Sprinkle the reserved mixture of cheese and onion on top before serving.

**Nutritional information:**

- Fat: 23 grams

- Carbohydrate: 34 grams

- Protein: 28 grams

# CASSEROLE WITH FLAVOUR FROM MEXICO

- Yield: 8

- Time taken: 4 hours 30 minutes

**Ingredients:**

- ✓ 1 lb. chorizo sausage

- ✓ 1½ cup milk

- ✓ 9 corn tortillas

- ✓ 8 eggs

- ✓ 1 red bell pepper, chopped

- ✓ 1 jalapeno chili, seeded and finely chopped

✓ 2 cups Pepper Jack cheese, shredded

✓ ¾ cup sliced green onions

✓ 2 tbsps. Fresh cilantro, chopped

✓ 1 cup Old El Paso salsa

**Directions:**

1. Coat the slow cooker with cooking spray and place 3 tortillas at the bottom. You may need to tear them to cover the bottom completely.

2. Mix eggs with milk in a bowl.

3. Remember to reserve 2 tablespoon of onions and ¾ cup cheese.

4. Top the tortillas with half portion of sausage followed by layers of green onion, bell peppers and cheese and repeat the layers with remaining ingredients.

5. Top the layering with the remaining tortillas and then pour the egg mixture from top.

6. Cover the cooker and cook on low setting for 4 hours making sure that the egg is set.

7. Sprinkle the cheese and onions before serving.

**Nutritional information:**

- Fat: 38 grams

- Carbohydrate: 20 grams

- Protein: 29 grams

## *FRENCH TOAST WITH APPLE FILLING*

- Yield: 8

- Time taken: 3 hours 5 minutes

**Ingredients:**

**For making French toast:**

- ✓ 8 eggs

- ✓ 10 cups of cubed French bread

- ✓ 2 cups of half-n-half

- ✓ 1/3 cup packed light brown sugar

- ✓ ½ cup milk

- ✓ 1½ tsp vanilla

- ✓ ½ tsp ground cinnamon

**For apple filling:**

- ✓ 3 apples, peeled and chopped coarsely

- ✓ 8 tbsps. Softened butter

- ✓ 1 cup packed light brown sugar

- ✓ 1 cup pecans, coarsely chopped

- ✓ 1 tsp ground cinnamon

**For topping:**

- ✓ Powdered sugar

- ✓ Maple syrup

**Directions:**

1. Keep the oven ready by preheating at 300 degrees and spread the bread cubes on a cookie sheet. Bake them for 20 minutes making sure that they become dry.

2. Line a slow cooker with a foil and coat it with cooking spray.

3. Use a bowl to mix the toast making ingredients and fold in the dried bread cubes in it. Allow standing time of 15 minutes, folding in between.

4. Melt 2 tablespoon butter in a skillet and cook the apples for 5 minutes with occasional stirring.

5. Use another bowl to mix the remaining 6 tablespoons of butter and remaining apple filling ingredients till they become crumbly.

6. Pour half portion of bread mixture in the slow cooker and top with apple filling and then sprinkle half portion of brown sugar and repeat the layering.

7. Cover the pot and cook for 3 hours on low setting until the center is set.

8. Sprinkle with powdered sugar and top with syrup.

Nutritional information:

- Fat: 35 grams

- Carbohydrate: 76 grams

- Protein: 15 grams

# CARAMEL ROLLS

- Serves: 4

- Prep time: 10 minutes

**Ingredients**

- ✓ 8 Refrigerator biscuits

- ✓ ½ cup brown sugar

- ✓ 4 tablespoons butter

**Directions**

1. Grease the Crockpot.

2. Place the biscuits right at the bottom of the crock pot.

3. In a pan, cook butter and brown sugar until the sugar melts. Pour over the biscuits.

4. Add some small pieces of nuts on the biscuit before cooking.

5. Cook for 1 hour on high.


# *SLOW COOKERBREAKFAST CASSEROLE*

- Serves: 8

- Prep time: 15 minutes

- Cook time: 4 hours on high/for 8 hours on low

## Ingredients

- ✓ 1 lb. bacon

- ✓ A dozen eggs

- ✓ 30 oz. frozen hash brown potatoes

- ✓ ½ red bell pepper, diced

- ✓ ½ medium green bell pepper, diced

- ✓ 1 medium onion, diced

- ✓ 8 oz. sharp cheddar cheese, shredded

- ✓ 1 cup milk

## Directions

1. Dice the bacon to small pieces.

2. The order in which things go in is:

- ½ the potatoes go in first

- ½ the bacon next

- ½ the onion next

- ½ the peppers next (both red and green)

- ½ the cheese next

- The other half of the potatoes

- The other half of the bacon

- The other half of the onion

- The other half of the peppers (both red and green)

- The other half of the cheese.

3. In a medium sized bowl beat eggs and milk together.

4. Pour egg mixture over your casserole.

5. Sprinkle salt and pepper on the ingredients.

6. Cook for 4 hours on high/for 8 hours on low

## *OVERNIGHT SLOW COOK CINNAMON APPLE*

- Serves: 6-8

- Prep time: 15 minutes

- Cook time: 5-7 hours on low

**Ingredients**

- ✓ 2 apples cored, peeled and diced

- ✓ 1 teaspoon cinnamon

- ✓ 1½ cups coconut milk

- ✓ 1 tablespoon coconut oil
- ✓ 1 tablespoon brown sugar
- ✓ 1 cup steel cut oats
- ✓ 1½ cups water
- ✓ ¼ teaspoon sea salt

## Directions

1. Grease the Crockpot.
2. Assemble all ingredients other than the toppings in the greased pot.
3. Cook for 5-7 hours on low.

# *SLOW COOKERBREAKFAST QUINOA*

## Ingredients

- ✓ 3 cups milk
- ✓ 1 cup quinoa
- ✓ 1 apple, peeled and diced
- ✓ ¼ cup pepitas
- ✓ 4 dates, chopped
- ✓ ¼ teaspoon nutmeg
- ✓ 2 teaspoon cinnamon
- ✓ 1 teaspoon vanilla extract
- ✓ ¼ teaspoon salt

## Directions

1. Assemble all the ingredients in the pot and cook on high for 2 hours. Make sure all the liquid is absorbed.

2. Cook on high for 2 hours or until all the liquid is absorbed.

3. You can cook this overnight as well. 8 hours on low for overnight cooking.

## SLOW COOK CREAMY COCONUT OATS

- Serves: 4

- Prep time: 10 minutes

- Cook time: 8 hours on low or 2 hours on high

**Ingredients**

- ✓ 2 cups steel cut oatmeal

- ✓ 1 can coconut milk, full fat

- ✓ 1 teaspoon vanilla

- ✓ 2 tablespoons organic cane sugar or coconut sugar

- ✓ 8 cups water

**Directions**

1. Assemble all the ingredients in the pot and cook on high for 2 hours. Make sure all the liquid is absorbed. You can also cook on low for 8 hours.

2. You have a lot of options to serve with. You can use coconut flakes, nut butter, raisins, pumpkin seeds, chia seeds, dried fruit, etc.

## BREAKFAST CROCKPOT OATMEAL

- Serves: 4

- Prep time: 10 minutes
- Cook time: 8 hours on low

## Ingredients

- ✓ 1 cup rolled oats
- ✓ 1 cup apple, chopped
- ✓ ½ cup raisins
- ✓ ½ cup walnuts, chopped
- ✓ ¼ cup brown sugar
- ✓ ½ teaspoon cinnamon
- ✓ 1 tablespoon butter, melted
- ✓ 2 cups milk
- ✓ ¼ teaspoon salt

## Directions

1. Apply nonstick spray inside the Crockpot.
2. Assemble all the products and whisk.
3. Cook for 8 hours on low

# *SLOW COOK BACON BREAKFAST*

- Serves: 10
- Prep time: 10 minutes
- Cook time: 10-12 hours on low

## Ingredients

- ✓ 1 lb. cooked bacon, drained and diced

- ✓ 30 oz. hash browns, frozen

- ✓ 12 eggs

- ✓ 1 cup milk

- ✓ ½ cup onion, diced

- ✓ ¾ pound shredded cheddar cheese

- ✓ ½ teaspoon dry mustard

- ✓ Salt

- ✓ Pepper

**Directions**

1. Layer the following in the order suggested:

- ½ the hash browns go in first

- ½ the bacon next

- ½ the onions next

- ½ the cheese next

- Rest of the hash browns

- Rest of the bacon

- Rest of the onions

- Rest of the cheese

2. Beat the eggs and mix them with mustard, milk, salt and pepper and pour over the layers.

3. Cook for 10-12 hours on low

## *CROCKPOT FRENCH TOAST CASSEROLE*

- Serves: 8

- Prep time: 10 minutes

- Cook time: low for 4 hours/high for 2 hours

## Ingredients

- ✓ 1 loaf of bread, sliced and quartered

- ✓ 6 eggs

- ✓ 2 cups milk

- ✓ ½ teaspoon cinnamon

- ✓ *For topping:*

- ✓ 1 teaspoon cinnamon

- ✓ ¼ cup butter

- ✓ ½ cup chopped pecans

- ✓ ½ cup firmly packed brown sugar

- ✓ A bit of nutmeg

## Directions

1. Mix and whisk the milk, eggs, and cinnamon and let the bread absorb that overnight or at least for 4 hours.

2. Grease the Crockpot and place the soaked bread in it.

3. Mix the ingredients for topping and sprinkle over the bread.

4. Cook on low for 4 hours or on high for 2 hours.


# *SLOW COOK TATER TOT EGG BAKE*

- Serves: 4

- Prep time: 15 minutes
- Cook time: 6-8 hours on low

**Ingredients**

- ✓ 6 oz. Canadian bacon, diced
- ✓ 2 onions, chopped
- ✓ 30 oz. Tater Tots
- ✓ ¼ cup Parmesan cheese, grated
- ✓ 2 cups cheddar cheese, shredded
- ✓ 4 Tablespoon all-purpose flour
- ✓ 12 eggs
- ✓ 1 cup milk
- ✓ 1 teaspoon salt
- ✓ ½ teaspoon pepper

**Directions**

1. Apply nonstick spray inside the pot.
2. Layer it in the order mentioned, *thrice*: 1/3 tots, 1/3 Canadian bacon, 1/3 onions and 1/3 cheese.
3. Whisk together the other ingredients and pour into the pot.
4. Cook for 6-8 hours on low

## *SLOW COOKER APPLE PIE OATMEAL*

- Serves: 4
- Prep time: 10 minutes

- Cook time: 7 hours on low

## Ingredients

- ✓ 3 small apples, cored, peeled and diced
- ✓ 1 cup steel cut oats
- ✓ 1 ½ cup almond milk, unsweetened
- ✓ 2 teaspoons cinnamon, ground
- ✓ 2 tablespoons hemp seeds
- ✓ ¼ teaspoon nutmeg, ground
- ✓ 1 teaspoon pure vanilla extract
- ✓ 2 tablespoons maple syrup
- ✓ 2 ½ cups water
- ✓ ¼ teaspoon salt

### *To top and serve:*

- ✓ Chopped pecans
- ✓ Raisins
- ✓ Almond Milk
- ✓ Maple syrup or brown sugar
- ✓ Ground cinnamon

## Directions

1. Grease the Crockpot.

2. Assemble and stir in all the ingredients and cook for 7 hours on low.

3. Before serving, stir in well and top it up with suggested ingredients or those of your choice

# CLASSIC BAKED APPLES

- Serves: 6

- Prep time: 30 minutes

- Cook time: 2 ½ to 3 ½ hours on high

**Ingredients:**

- ✓ 6 medium baking apples, cored

- ✓ 2 tablespoons golden raisins

- ✓ ¼ cup orange juice

- ✓ 1 teaspoon lemon juice

- ✓ 1 teaspoon ground cinnamon

- ✓ 2 tablespoons butter

- ✓ ¼ cup dark brown sugar, packed

- ✓ ¼ cup water

**Directions:**

1. Mix in the raisins, lemon juice, and sugar to make a filling and stuff the cored apples with it.

2. Arrange the apples in the pot and sprinkle with cinnamon and butter. Pour the orange juice over the apples.

3. Cook for 2 ½ to 3 ½ hours on high.

4. Serve the apples topped with the sauce remaining in the pot

# APPLE CONFIT DELIGHT

- Serves: 8

- Prep time: 20 minutes

- Cook time: 4 – 4 ½ hours on low

**Ingredients:**

- ✓ 3 lbs. Golden Delicious or Granny Smith apples

- ✓ ½ teaspoon ground cinnamon

- ✓ 1 teaspoon real vanilla extract

- ✓ ¼ cup light brown sugar

**Directions:**

1. Peel the apples and slice to ¼ inch thickness. Drizzle the cinnamon and brown sugar over the apples and coat the apples properly.

2. Cook for 4 – 4 ½ hours on low.

3. Stir in the vanilla and mix properly

# SWEET & TANGY ORANGEADE

- Serves: 10

- Prep time: 15 minutes

- Cook time: 3 hours on low

**Ingredients:**

- ✓ 1 ½ cups of orange juice

- ✓ ¼ cups of pineapple juice

- ✓ 3/4 cups of lemon juice

- ✓ ½ teaspoon of cloves

- ✓ 1 large cinnamon stick

- ✓ 2 cups of sugar

- ✓ 2 ½ quarts of water

**Directions:**

1. In a Crockpot, mix (in the order mentioned): water, then stir in the sugar, then the orange juice, then the lemon juice, and finally the pineapple juice. Mix well.

2. Place the cinnamon stick and cloves into a double layer cheesecloth bag, tie the top and place into the crock pot.

3. Cook for 3 hours on low.

4. Dispose of the cheesecloth bag before you serve

## *SLOW COOK SIMMERED ALMOND TEA*

- Serves: 10

- Prep time: 15 minutes

- Cook time: 1 hour on high

**Ingredients:**

- ✓ 1 tablespoon instant tea

- ✓ 2/3 cups of lemon juice

- ✓ 1 teaspoon vanilla

- ✓ 1 teaspoon almond extract

- ✓ 6 tablespoon sugar

- ✓ 10 cups of boiling water

**Directions:**

1. Pour in the water into the Crockpot. Add and dissolve the tea, then the lemon juice, then the sugar, then the vanilla and finally the almond extract. Mix well.

2. Cook for 1 hour on high

# WHIPPED UP CHOCOLATE COFFEE

- Serves: 4

- Prep time: 15 minutes

- Cook time: 3 hours on low

**Ingredients:**

- ✓ 3 tablespoon chocolate syrup

- ✓ 3 cups of strong coffee

- ✓ ¼ cups of crème de cacao

- ✓ 1/3 cups of heavy whipping cream

- ✓ 1 teaspoon sugar

**Directions:**

1. The coffee goes into the Crockpot first. Add and mix the chocolate syrup and sugar.

2. Cook for 150 minutes on low.

3. Stir in the whipping cream and crème de cacao.

4. Cook for another 30 minutes on low

# BACON, HASH BROWN & EGG CASSEROLE

- Serves: 6

- Prep time: 20 minutes

- Cook time: 2-3 hours on high

**Ingredients:**

- ✓ 20 oz. hash browns, shredded, frozen and thawed

- ✓ 8 slices of thick-cut bacon, coarsely chopped and cooked

- ✓ 6 sliced thin green onions

- ✓ 8 oz. cheddar cheese, shredded

- ✓ ½ cup milk

- ✓ 12 eggs

- ✓ ½ teaspoon salt

- ✓ ¼ teaspoon pepper

**Directions**

1. Grease the Crockpot.

2. Layer half of the hash browns at the bottom of the crockpot, followed by a layer of half the cheese and then a layer of half the bacon at the top. Add in 1/3 of the green onions.

3. Put aside some green onions and bacon for garnish.

4. Repeat the second layer as in the first i.e. layer hash browns followed by bacon then cheese and finally onions.

5. Whisk together milk, eggs, pepper and salt in a large bowl.

6. Pour over the top (of the ingredients in the crockpot), slowly.

7. Cook for 2-3 hours on high until the eggs are set.

8. Sprinkle with some more bacons and onions, then serve

# BLUEBERRY CREAM CHEESE PUDDING

- Serves: 8

- Prep time: 20 minutes

- Cook time: 4-5 hours on low

**Ingredients:**

- ✓ 2 cups fresh or frozen blueberries

- ✓ 1 tablespoon vanilla extract

- ✓ 8 oz. cream cheese, cut into 1 inch cubes

- ✓ 5 eggs

- ✓ 4 cups whole milk

- ✓ 1 tablespoon cinnamon

- ✓ ¾ cup maple syrup

- ✓ 8 cups bread, cubed

**Directions:**

1. Mix eggs and milk in a bowl and whisk. Add vanilla, cinnamon and maple syrup. Stir in the bread. Let it be for 20 minutes.

2. Grease your Crockpot.

3. Mix in the blueberries and cream cheese.

4. Cook in the Crockpot for 4-5 hours on low


# SLOW COOK GRANOLA APPLES

- Serves: 4

- Prep time: 15 minutes

- Cook time: 4-5 hours on low

**Ingredients:**

- ✓ 4 medium-sized Gala apples
- ✓ 4 teaspoons maple syrup
- ✓ ½ cup granola
- ✓ 1 tablespoons melted butter
- ✓ Whipped cream, for serving

**Directions:**

1. Using a knife, cut off a layer on top pf the apples.
2. Use a spoon to remove the seeds and core from the apples. Stuff each apple with an eighth cup of granola.
3. Place gently into the SLOW COOKER the sprinkle butter over the apples and add a spoonful of maple syrup over each.
4. Cook for 4-5 hours on low or until tender.
5. Top with whipped cream when serving

## *SLOW COOKERFRENCH TOAST*

- Serves: 6
- Prep time: 15 minutes
- Cook time: 6 hours on low

**Ingredients:**

- ✓ ½ loaf of bread
- ✓ 6 eggs

- ✓ 2 cups milk

- ✓ 1 teaspoon cinnamon

- ✓ 1 teaspoon vanilla.

- ✓ 1 tablespoon light brown sugar

**Directions:**

1. Mix all ingredients other than the bread and soak the bread in the mixture.

2. Cook for 6 hours on low

# *SLOW COOKERBREAKFAST RISOTTO*

- Serves: 3

- Prep time: 15 minutes

- Cook time: 3-5 hours on high

**Ingredients:**

- ✓ ¼ cup butter

- ✓ 3 small apples

- ✓ 1/8 teaspoon cloves

- ✓ 1/8 teaspoon nutmeg

- ✓ 1 ½ teaspoon cinnamon

- ✓ 1 ½ cups Arborio rice

- ✓ ¼ teaspoon kosher salt

- ✓ 1/3 cup brown sugar

- ✓ 4 cups of apple juice

**Directions:**

1. Grease the Crockpot with butter. Slice the apples and add them in.

2. Stir in to coat the apples with the other ingredients.

3. Cook on high for 3-5 hours.

# SLOW COOKER BREADS AND SANDWICHES

What's different about the variety of breads available today is that cooks around the globe are getting very creative with the combination of ingredients they incorporate. Because SLOW COOKER breads are nearly impossible to burn, bakers of all experience levels are donning their chef's hats and getting in on the action. After all, what's more enticing than strolling into your home than being met by the welcoming aroma of hot, fresh bread?

**Tip 35:** Always spray, butter or line baking dishes or SLOW COOKER inserts with parchment. Silicone works, too.

**Tip 36:** Keep heavy ingredients such as fruit, nuts and vegetables from sinking to the bottom of your loaves by dusting with a smidge of flour before adding to the batter.

**Tip 37:** Avoid over-mixing to refrain from having loaves with large tunnels and voids.

**Tip 38:** Thickness plays a part in the length of time bread needs to bake. The larger, thicker loaves need more time in order to be cooked throughout.

**Tip 39:** Over-mixing batter and dough cause's quick breads to be tough, so does being baked in too high a temperature.

**Tip 40:** Too much liquid leads to soggy bread, while too much fat leads to loaves with extra-crisp edges.

**Tip 41:** Though it's true that salt adds flavor, it also controls how much the yeast grows, ensuring loaves won't rise too high. It's especially important in quick breads that have oodles of sugar on which yeast feeds.

**Tip 42:** SLOW COOKER cooking is a breeze! Even your first loaf of bread will make you a star because *nothing* burns when cooked on LOW heat. Breads have a nice crust; meats are juicy and tender.

**Tip 43:** Convert any recipe to cook in a crock pot, even those written for bread machines work very nicely. Typically, you'd reduce liquids by about a third--or add 1/2 cup water if a recipe calls for none. It also helps to increase timing. Cooking foods on HIGH heat takes half as long as cooking on LOW heat. Use this handy chart to help convert cooking times and temperatures:

| Oven / Stove top | LOW Heat (200 C.) | HIGH Heat (300 C.) |
|---|---|---|
| 15 to 30 minutes | 4 to 6 hours | 1 1/2 to 2 1/2 hours |
| 35 to 45 minutes | 6 to 8 hours | 3 to 4 hours |
| 50 minutes to 3 hours | 8 to 10 hours | 4 to 6 hours |

**Tip 44:** Keep an eye on your bread during baking so it does not get overdone. Using a SLOW COOKER with a white ceramic insert lends best results.

**Tip 45:** Quick breads bake best when mixed least. Be sure to aerate combined dry ingredients before adding to liquids. Don't worry if there are lumps as most disappear during baking.

## BREAD IN A CROCKPOT

- Yield: App 1 lb. loaf

- Time taken: 2 hours

**Ingredients:**

- ✓ 1 tbsp. granulated yeast

- ✓ 3 cups of warm water

- ✓ 975 grams of plain flour

- ✓ 1 tbsp. salt

**Directions:**

1. Put salt, yeast and water in a container and whisk them together. Add the flour and use a wooden spoon to combine all the ingredients.

2. Cover the container loosely with cloth and leave for 2 hours so that the dough can rise.

3. Sprinkle some flour over the dough and put it on a sheet of baking paper.

4. Now, sprinkle the top of the dough with flour and place it in the crockpot.

5. Cook on low settings for 2 hours and serve by slicing.

## *CROCKPOT BREAD WITH SHORTENING*

- Yield: Approximately ½ lb.

- Time taken: 2 hours 30 minutes

**Ingredients:**

- ✓ 1¼ cups of warm water

- ✓ 0.25 oz. active dry yeast

- ✓ ½ tbsp. salt

- ✓ 1½ tbsp. sugar

- ✓ 1 tbsp. shortening

- ✓ 3 cups of unbleached bread flour

**Directions:**

1. Dissolve yeast in warm water and allow standing time of 10 minutes.

2. Now add sugar, salt and shortening and when they are properly mixed, start adding the flour. Use a wooden spoon to make a smooth paste.

3. Line the crockpot with a parchment paper and roll the dough to form a ball so that it can be easily placed in the pot.

4. Cook on low setting for 2 hours 15 minutes and then allow cooling on a wire rack.

# APPLE PIE BREAD

- Serves:16

- Prep. Time:10 minutes

- Cook time:1 hour

**Ingredients**

- ✓ 1 cup flour

- ✓ 1 1/2 teaspoons baking powder

- ✓ 1/2 teaspoon salt

- ✓ 1/2 cup milk

- ✓ 1 Tablespoon butter, melted

- ✓ 1 egg

- ✓ 1 cup of Apple Pie Filling

**Directions**

1. Combine dry ingredients; add milk, butter and egg, blending well.

2. By hand, add pie filling by spoonful, folding in gently.

3. Transfer to pot, spreading carefully so mixture flattens evenly.

4. Cover; cook on HIGH for 1 hour. Test doneness by inserting tester near center; if comes out clean, gently slide knife about edges to loosen loaf, then transfer to rack to cool before slicing (or serve warm, straight from the pot).

# APPLESAUCE BREAD

- Serves:8 to 12

- Prep. Time:10 minutes

- Cook Time:8 hours

Spray or butter baking dish or crock insert.

## Ingredients

- ✓ 1/2 cup butter, melted
- ✓ 1 cup sugar
- ✓ 2 eggs
- ✓ 1 t. vanilla
- ✓ 2 cups flour
- ✓ 1 t. baking powder
- ✓ 1 t. salt
- ✓ 1/2 teaspoon baking soda
- ✓ 1/2 teaspoon cinnamon
- ✓ 1/2 teaspoon nutmeg
- ✓ 1 1/4 cup applesauce
- ✓ 1/2 cup pecans, optional

## Directions

1. Whisk together dry ingredients, set aside.

2. Cream sugar with shortening till light, mix in eggs and vanilla.

3. Add half dry ingredients, mixing well. Follow with applesauce and remaining dry mixture, stir until just combined.

4. Spread in container; bake on LOW heat for 8 hours (or HIGH for 4 hours). Turn off heat; let stand 10 minutes before transferring to wire rack to cool and glaze.

# BLUEBERRY COFFEE-CAKE BREAD

- Serves:8

- Prep. Time:5 minutes

- Cook Time:4 hours

Spray or butter crock insert.

## Ingredients

- ✓ 2 large eggs

- ✓ 1/2 cup sugar

- ✓ 1/2 cup brown sugar, packed firmly

- ✓ 2/3 cup butter, melted

- ✓ 1 teaspoon vanilla

- ✓ 1 teaspoon cinnamon

- ✓ 2 cups biscuit mix (gluten-free baking mix works well, too)

- ✓ 1 cup sour cream

- ✓ 1/2 cup frozen blueberries

## Directions

1. Cream eggs and sugar, add butter, vanilla and cinnamon.

2. Reduce speed, alternate adding biscuit mix and sour cream, combining well.

3. Gently fold in fruit; spread batter in crock. Cover with lid set slightly ajar using wooden skewer. Bake on HIGH heat, 2 to 4 hours, until a tester inserted near center comes out clean.

# *BUTTERMILK, BRAN & CHEDDAR BREAD*

- Serves:12

- Prep. Time:10 minutes

- Cook Time:4 to 6 hours

- Spray or butter baking dish.

## Ingredients

- ✓ 1 cup whole bran

- ✓ 1 1/4 cups buttermilk or sour milk

- ✓ 1 1/2 cups flour

- ✓ 1 1/2 teaspoons baking powder

- ✓ 1/4 teaspoon baking soda

- ✓ 1/2 teaspoon salt

- ✓ 1/3 cup sugar

- ✓ 1/4 cup shortening

- ✓ 1 egg

- ✓ 1 cup Shredded Sharp Cheddar Cheese

## Directions

1. Let bran soften in milk; set aside.

2. Lightly whisk dry ingredients; set aside.

3. Cream sugar and lard until fluffy; beat in egg. Alternately add dry ingredients and milk mixture, combining well after each addition. Gently fold in cheese, then spread batter in crock.

4. Bake on LOW heat 4 to 6 hours (or on HIGH for 2 to 3 hours), until tester comes out clean. Slide knife about pan edges gently to loosen loaf; transfer bread to wire rack to cool completely

# CHOCOLATE GUINNESS LOAF

- Serves:12

- Prep. Time:15 minutes

- Cook time:4 hours


- Butter or spray sides and bottom of baking dish or crock insert.

**Ingredients**

- ✓ 1 1/2 cups flour

- ✓ 1/2 cup cocoa powder

- ✓ 1 teaspoon salt

- ✓ 1 teaspoon baking soda

- ✓ 2 cubes unsalted butter, melted

- ✓ 1 1/2 cups packed light brown sugar

- ✓ 2 large eggs

- ✓ 1 teaspoon Pure Vanilla extract

- ✓ 1 cup Guinness

✓ 1 cup semisweet chocolate chips

**Directions**

1. Combine first 4 ingredients, whisking lightly; set aside.

2. Cream butter and sugar; add eggs and vanilla. Alternate small additions of flour mixture and Guinness, mixing well after each. When smooth, fold in chips and spread evenly in baking dish.

3. Bake on LOW heat for 8 hours (or on HIGH for 4 hours), until tester inserted near center comes out clean. Turn off heat; let stand 10 minutes before inverting to wire rack to cool completely. Store leftovers in airtight container, though it's unlikely any will be left.

# *CINNAMON-VANILLA FRENCH TOAST*

- Serves: 12 to 16

- Prep. Time: 10 minutes

- Cook time: 2:40 to 4:40 hours, divided plus 20 minutes standing time

- Prepare SLOW COOKER insert with generous layer of cooking spray or butter.

- Preheat traditional oven to 220 degrees.

**Ingredients**

✓ Cooking spray or butter to grease the crockpot

✓ 1 loaf French bread, torn or cut in 1-inch cubes

✓ 8 eggs

✓ 1 teaspoons vanilla

✓ 2 teaspoons cinnamon

✓ 1 cup French Vanilla creamer

- ✓ 2.5 cups 2% (or richer) milk

- ✓ 1/4 cup brown sugar

- ✓ 4 Tablespoons butter, softened

- ✓ 2 cups chopped walnuts or pecans

**Directions**

1. Bake cubed bread in jelly roll pan (lip saves any pieces that wander) or on cookie sheets at 220 degrees, 30 to 40 minutes, until bread is dried out. Transfer to pot insert; set aside.

2. Beat eggs, spices and liquids; pour over bread, pushing cubes down until mixture soaks into it.

3. Combine remaining 3 ingredients well; gently fold into bread mixture.

4. Cover; cook on LOW heat for 4 hours (or HIGH heat for 2 hours), until center of French toast is set but moist. Then turn heat OFF and let stand 15 to 20 minutes, uncovered.

5. Plate; serve sprinkled with powdered sugar or drizzled with maple syrup.

# CITRUS MARMALADE LOAF

- Serves: 12

- Prep. Time: 20 minutes

- Cook Time: 55 minutes

- Spray baking dish or crock insert.

**Ingredients**

- ✓ 1 1/2 cups flour

- ✓ 1 1/2 teaspoons baking powder

- ✓ 1 teaspoon salt

- ✓ 4 Tablespoons powdered sugar

- ✓ 2/3 cup lemon marmalade, divided

- ✓ 1 cup unsalted butter, softened

- ✓ 3/4 cup sugar

- ✓ 2 teaspoons grated lemon zest

- ✓ 1 teaspoon grated orange zest

- ✓ 3 large eggs, room temperature

- ✓ 2 Tablespoons freshly squeezed orange juice

## Directions

1. Combine first 4 ingredients in separate bowl; set aside. Check jam for oddly large hunks of peel; chop so about 1 inch in size, set aside.

2. Cream butter, sugar and zest until fluffy; beat in eggs one at a time.

3. Add juice and half the jam. Reduce speed, add dry ingredients in smallish batches, beating until just combined.

4. Spread batter in pan; bake on LOW heat for 6 to 8 hours (or on HIGH for 3 to 4 hours), until top of loaf is golden brown and tester comes out clean.

5. Transfer pan to wire rack and with bread still inside, let stand 10 minutes before inverting loaf onto rack to cool completely.

GLAZE

1. Warm remaining jam over medium heat; then stir in sugar and 1/2 Tablespoon butter until smooth.

2. Pour over top of cooled cake.

# CONFETTI BREAD

- Serves:12 to 16

- Prep. Time:10 minutes

- Cook time:8 hours

## Ingredients

- ✓ 1 3/4 cup flour

- ✓ 1 1/2 cup sugar

- ✓ 1 teaspoon baking soda

- ✓ 1/2 teaspoon salt

- ✓ 1 teaspoon cinnamon

- ✓ 1/2 teaspoon nutmeg

- ✓ 2 eggs

- ✓ 1 cup ripe banana, mashed

- ✓ 1/2 cup vegetable oil

- ✓ 1/3 cup buttermilk or sour milk

- ✓ 1 teaspoon Pure Vanilla

- ✓ 1/2 cup dried fruit*

- ✓ 1/2 cup pecans, chopped

- ✓ 1/2 cup chocolate chips

## Directions

1. Combine dry ingredients; whisk, set aside.

2. Beat eggs, blend in banana and liquids. Reduce speed, mix in dry ingredients, a cup at a time, beating well. Fold in dried fruit, chocolate and nuts.

3. Spread in baking dish, cover and bake on LOW heat for 8 hours (or on HIGH for 4 hours), until tester inserted near center comes out clean.

4. Let stand, uncovered, 10 minutes. Gently slide knife around edges of container; transfer to wire rack to cool completely.

5. Once completely cooled, store in airtight container 8 or more hours before enjoying, so flavors have a chance to meld.

# SWEDISH BUTTERMILK CRANBERRY BREAD

- Serves:12

- Prep. Time:5 minutes

- Cook Time:8 to 10 hours

- Spray or butter crock insert or baking bowl.

**Ingredients**

- ✓ 2 cups buttermilk

- ✓ 1 (14 ounce) can whole cranberry sauce

- ✓ 1 cup flaxseed

- ✓ 1/2 cup hazelnuts, chopped

- ✓ 1/2 cup sunflower seeds

- ✓ 1/2 cup pumpkin seeds

- ✓ 1 cup rolled oats or oat bran

- ✓ 1 1/2 teaspoons baking soda

- ✓ 1 1/2 teaspoons baking soda

- ✓ 1 teaspoon coarse salt

- ✓ 1 cup wheat germ

- ✓ 2 1/2 cups whole wheat flour

**Directions**

1. Combine dry ingredients, whisk lightly; set aside.

2. Blend milk and sauce; beat in small amounts of dry mixture, combining well.

3. Spread batter in pan and cook, uncovered, on LOW for 8 to 10 hours (or HIGH for 4 to 6 hours), until tester inserted near center comes out clean.

## *SLOW COOK GUMDROP BREAD*

- Serves:12

- Prep. Time:10 minutes

- Cook time:8 to 10 hours

**Ingredients**

- ✓ 2 1/2 cups flour

- ✓ 1/2 cup sugar

- ✓ 1/2 cup brown sugar, packed

- ✓ 1/4 cup shortening

- ✓ 1 1/4 cups buttermilk

- ✓ 3 teaspoons baking powder

- ✓ 1 teaspoon salt

- ✓ 1 teaspoon vanilla

- ✓ 1/2 teaspoon baking soda

- ✓ 2 eggs

- ✓ 1 cup small gumdrop, halved

- ✓ 1/2 cup nuts, chopped (optional)

## Directions

1. Mix all ingredients but nuts and candy; then fold those in and combine well.

2. Spread mixture in pan and bake on LOW heat 8 hours (or on HIGH for 4 hours), until tester comes out clean. Run knife about edges of loaf to loosen, then transfer bread to cool completely on wire rack.

3. Slice and refrigerate in airtight container 8 to 12 hours prior to serving.

# *JUNGLE BREAD*

- Serves:12

- Prep. Time:20 minutes

- Cook time:1:55 hours

- Spray or butter 4 1/2- to 5-quart crock.

## Ingredients (Bread)

- ✓ 1 cube butter

- ✓ 2/3 cup brown sugar, packed

- ✓ 1/4 cup sugar

- ✓ 1 (16.3 ounce) tube refrigerated Buttermilk biscuits, quartered

- ✓ 3/4 cup pecan halves

## Directions

1. Combine sugar and quartered dough in baggy and shake to coat.

2. Cream butter and sugar; heat in microwave 2 minutes, stirring every 30 seconds, until mixture is smooth and boiling.

3. Layer bottom of crock with a third of the nuts. Arrange half the biscuits over nuts, then pour a third of the sugar syrup over them.

4. Repeat first 2 layers again, then cover with remaining 2/3 syrup and top with remaining nuts.

5. Cover; cook on HIGH 2 to 3 hours, until tester comes out clean and center not doughy. Be aware, though, that top will appear unbaked.

6. Turn heat off and remove lid carefully so condensation does *not* drip onto bread. Lightly cover opening with paper towels, then return lid over pot and let stand 10 minutes.

7. Gently loosen edges of bread, running knife about before inverting on heat-resistant serving platter to cool. Make sauce.

## Ingredients (Jungle Sauce)

✓ 2 Tablespoons whipping cream, un-whipped

✓ 1/3 cup milk chocolate chips OR 1/4 hot fudge sauce

## Directions

1. Heat cream over medium heat until tiny bubbles appear around edges.

2. Remove from heat; stir in chips until mixture is smooth.

3. Drizzle over loaf in any pattern. Serve warm with gobs of cold milk.

# CHOCOLATE BANANA BREAD

- Serves:12

- Prep. Time:20 minutes

- Cook Time: 3 1/2 to 4 1/2 hours

- Ideal in 6-quart crock pot. Be sure to spray or butter baking dish.

## Ingredients

- ✓ 2 cups flour

- ✓ 3/4 teaspoon baking soda

- ✓ 1/2 teaspoon salt

- ✓ 1 cup (3 medium) over-ripe bananas, mashed

- ✓ 1/2 cup creamy peanut butter

- ✓ 1/2 cup sugar

- ✓ 2 large eggs

- ✓ 1/3 cup buttermilk

- ✓ 1/3 cup vegetable oil

- ✓ 1 teaspoon vanilla

- ✓ 1 cup semisweet chocolate chips

## Directions

1. Combine first 3 ingredients; set aside.

2. Cream fruit and peanut butter; blend in next 5 items. Add dry ingredients, mixing smooth. Fold in chips.

3. Spread batter in whatever size baking dish fits your crock pot. Center on trivet or canning jar ring placed in center of crock.

4. Cover, propping lid slightly ajar with chopstick and bake on HIGH heat for 3½–4½ hours, until tester comes out clean. Turn off heat; don

heat-resistant gloves and carefully remove hot pan to cooling rack. Let stand 10 minutes. Gently slide knife about edge of loaf to loosen, then invert on wire rack to cool completely. Slices easily once cooled. Store in airtight container.

# *SMOKED CHEDDAR LOAF*

- Serves:16

- Prep. Time:15 minutes

- Cook Time:8 to 10 hours

## Ingredients

- ✓ 1 teaspoon active dry yeast

- ✓ 1/4 water, warmed

- ✓ 1 egg

- ✓ 1 Tablespoon sugar

- ✓ 3/4 cup mild-flavored beer

- ✓ 1 1/4 cups shredded Smoked Cheddar Cheese

- ✓ 3 cups flour

- ✓ 3/4 teaspoon salt

## Directions

1. Dissolve yeast in 1/4 cup warm water; set aside.

2. Cream egg and sugar. Add flour and salt, beat well. Reduce speed; alternately add small amounts of cheese and beer, combining well after each addition.

3. Spread in crock; cover and bake on LOW heat for 8 to 10 hours (or on HIGH for 4 to 6 hours), until tester comes out clean.

4. Slide knife around edges to loosen bread, then transfer to wire rack to cool completely.

# SOUR CREAM BANANA BREAD

- ✓ Serves:12

- ✓ Prep. Time:5 minutes

- ✓ Cook time:6 to 8 hours

- ✓ Butter or spray crock insert or straight-sided container.

## Ingredients

- ✓ 1 2/3 cups flour

- ✓ 1 teaspoon baking soda

- ✓ 1/2 teaspoon ground cinnamon

- ✓ 1/2 teaspoon salt

- ✓ 2 eggs

- ✓ 1/2 cup sugar

- ✓ 3/4 cup brown sugar

- ✓ 2 Tablespoons sour cream

- ✓ 1/2 cup vegetable oil

- ✓ 3 1/2 bananas (over-ripe), mashed

- ✓ 1 teaspoon vanilla extract

## Directions

1. Lightly whisk dry ingredients; set aside.

2. Cream eggs and sugar until fluffy; blend in cream, oil, vanilla, and fruit. Reduce mixer speed; beat in small amounts of dry mixture at a time, combining well after each.

3. Spread batter in pan; bake on LOW heat, 6 to 8 hours (or on HIGH for 3 to 4 hours), until crust is golden and tester comes out clean. (If top browns too fast, simply add loose cover over bread.)

4. Transfer to wire rack to cool completely. Store leftovers in airtight container.

# SPEEDY SAUSAGE LOAF

- Serves:12

- Prep. Time:15 minutes

- Cook Time:4 to 6 hours

- Spray baking dish or use flat silicone tray.

## Ingredients

- ✓ 3 Tablespoons butter

- ✓ 1 medium onion, chopped finely

- ✓ 2 large peppers, chopped finely

- ✓ 1 teaspoon garlic powder

- ✓ 1 pound sausage, *not* links

- ✓ 1 loaf frozen bread dough, thawed

## Directions

1. Melt butter; add veggies and sauté until onions are translucent.

2. Stir in garlic; add meat to brown. Drain excess oil.

3. On prepared pan, unroll dough. Spread meat mixture down center, then draw up sides and pinch ends.

4. Bake on LOW heat about 6 hours. Remove; top with butter and serve.

## *SLOW COOK SPOTTED DOG*

- Serves:8 to 10

- Prep. Time:5 minutes

- Cook Time:8 hours

- Spray or butter baking dish.

**Ingredients**

- ✓ 3 cups of all-purpose flour

- ✓ 1 teaspoon salt

- ✓ 1 teaspoon baking soda

- ✓ 1 tablespoon baking powder

- ✓ ⅔ Cup sugar

- ✓ 1 ½ cups raisins

- ✓ 2 large beaten eggs

- ✓ 3 teaspoons of caraway seeds

- ✓ 2 tablespoons salted butter, melted

- ✓ 2 cups buttermilk

- ✓ Softened butter for serving

**Directions**

1. Combine flour, sugar, salt, baking powder, and baking soda. Stir in raisins and seeds.

2. Create well in center of mixture; add wet ingredients and stir until combined.

3. Spread dough in prepared pan; bake on LOW heat for 8 hours (or on HIGH for 4 hours), until crust becomes golden brown and tester inserted near center comes out clean. Turn off heat; let stand 5 minutes before inverting bread onto wire rack to cool completely.

# TURTLE BREAD

- Serves: 12

- Prep. Time: 10 minutes

- Cook time: 3:30 hours

- Spray or butter baking dish or crock insert.

## Ingredients

✓ 1 1/2 teaspoons quick active dry yeast

✓ 1/4 cup lukewarm water

✓ 1 cup water

✓ 10 caramels, melted

✓ 2 2/3 cups bread flour

✓ 2 Tablespoons dry milk

✓ 1 Tablespoon sugar

✓ 3/4 teaspoon salt

✓ 1/4 cup semisweet chocolate chips

✓ 1/2 cup pecans, coarsely chopped

## Directions

1. Dissolve yeast in lukewarm water; set aside.

2. Whisk first 4 ingredients; blend in water, yeast mixture and melted candy until smooth. Fold in nuts and chips. Spread in pan.

3. Cover; bake on LOW heat, 8 hours (or on HIGH for 4 hours), until tester comes out clean. Transfer to wire rack to cool, but steel yourself if, when you return to slice it, you discover this turtle's gone.

## *WILD RICE BREAD*

- Serves: 16 to 20

- Prep. Time: 20 minutes

- Cook Time: 8 hours

## Instructions

- ✓ 1 packet active dry yeast

- ✓ 1/3 cup warm water

- ✓ 4 1/2 cup flour

- ✓ 2 cups whole wheat flour

- ✓ 1/2 cup rye flour

- ✓ 1/2 cup rolled oats

- ✓ 2 teaspoons salt

- ✓ 2 cup milk, scalded, cooled to 105 to 115 degrees

- ✓ 1/2 cup honey

- ✓ 2 Tablespoon butter, melted

- ✓ 1 cup wild rice, cooked

- ✓ 1 egg

✓ 1/4 cup cold water

**Directions**

1. Dissolve yeast in warm water; set aside.

2. Combine dry ingredients; set aside.

3. Blend liquids along with butter; pour in yeast, then mix in small amounts of dry ingredients, beating well after each addition. Fold in rice and enough additional flour to form stiff dough.

4. Transfer to lightly-floured surface to knead dough until elastic yet smooth, 8 to 10 minutes.

5. Put in greased bowl, turning once to grease top. Cover lightly with kitchen towel and place in warm spot to rise, 90 minutes.

6. Once doubled in size, punch down dough and return to lightly-floured surface. Divide in three sections, shape each into long even ropes.

7. Braid together, forming circle. Place in prepared vessel, cover and let rise until doubled again, 30 minutes.

8. Using fork, beat egg with cold water in small cup; dip pastry brush and lightly coat braided loaf.

9. Cover crock and bake on LOW heat for 7 to 8 hours (or on HIGH for 3 1/2 to 4 hours), until golden brown.

10. Transfer braid to wire rack to cool completely.

# WINE-A-ROUND BREAD

- Serves:48

- Prep. Time:15 minutes

- Cook time:4 to 6 hours

- Chill Time:2 hours

- Butter or spray flat silicone baking sheet.

**Ingredients**

- ✓ 1 packet yeast

- ✓ 1/4 cup water, warmed

- ✓ 4 cups flour

- ✓ 6 Tablespoons sugar

- ✓ 1 teaspoon salt

- ✓ 1 cup butter

- ✓ 4 yolks

- ✓ 1 cup warm milk

- ✓ 4 (30 ounce) cans fruit pie filling, different flavors (cherry, apple, blueberry, apricot )

**Directions**

1. Dissolve yeast in warm water; set aside.

2. Combine dry ingredients; cut in butter, as for traditional pie crust.

3. Beat yolks, blend in milk and yeast mixture. Slowly add flour, forming a sticky dough. Place in greased bowl, chill in refrigerator at least 2 hours.

4. Divide dough into fourths. Roll each quarter into long rectangles, about 1/4-inch thick, then shape into ring, sealing to hide ends.

5. Spread various fillings along center of dough, alternating at different intervals; then bring up both sides of dough, pinching to cover filling.

6. Bake in SLOW COOKER on LOW heat for 4 to 6 hours (or on HIGH for 2 to 3 hours).

7. Transfer to heat-resistant serving platter to cool. Store in airtight container.

# ZUCCHINI APPLESAUCE BREAD

- Serves: 12

- Prep. Time: 10 minutes

- Cook time: 8 hours

- Spray or butter straight-edged container, insert or baking bowl.

**Ingredients**

- ✓ 2 cups flour

- ✓ 1 1/2 teaspoons baking soda

- ✓ 3/4 teaspoon baking powder

- ✓ 1 teaspoon coarse salt

- ✓ 3 1/2 teaspoons cinnamon

- ✓ 3 eggs, room temperature

- ✓ 1/2 cup vegetable oil

- ✓ 1/2 cup plain applesauce

- ✓ 2 teaspoons Pure Vanilla extract

- ✓ 2 cups zucchini, freshly grated

- ✓ 1 1/2 cups sugar

**Directions**

1. Combine dry ingredients; set aside.

2. Beat eggs; blend oil, fruit, and vanilla. Add zucchini, then sugar, mixing well.

3. Reduce mixer speed to low; add dry ingredient mixture slowly, beating until completely combined after each addition.

4. Pour batter into prepared insert; cover and cook 8 hours on LOW (or 4 hours on HIGH) heat. Bread is done if center springs back when lightly touched.

# *PORK SUBWAY SANDWICH*

- Yield: 16

- Time taken: 5 hours 15 minutes

**Ingredients:**

- ✓ 2½ lb. boneless pork shoulder

- ✓ 1 small onion, finely chopped

- ✓ ¼ cup honey

- ✓ 18 oz. barbecue sauce

- ✓ ½ cup water

- ✓ 1 tsp seasoned salt

- ✓ 8 submarine buns

- ✓ 1 tsp ground ginger

- ✓ 6 garlic cloves, minced

**Directions:**

1. Roast the onions in a SLOW COOKER and then combine with barbecue sauce, honey, garlic, ginger and salt and pour it along with the meat in the cooker.

2. Cook on high setting for 5 hours.

3. Allow cooling and then shred the meat to place the required portions in the sandwiches.

**Nutritional information:**

- Fat: 13 grams

- Carbohydrate: 44 grams

- Protein: 29 grams

# *BBQ FLAVORED SANDWICH FROM A SLOW COOKER*

- Yield: 8

- Time taken: 4 hours 25 minutes

**Ingredients:**

**For brine:**

- ✓ ¼ cup packed brown sugar

- ✓ 1½ quarts water

- ✓ 2 tbsps. salt

- ✓ 2 garlic cloves, minced

- ✓ 1 tbsp. liquid smoke

- ✓ ½ tsp dried thyme

**For chicken:**

- ✓ 1/3 cup liquid smoke

- ✓ 2 lb. boneless chicken breast

- ✓ 1½ cup smoke flavored barbecue sauce

✓ 16 slider buns

**Directions:**

1. Mix the brine making ingredients in a bowl and stir the mixture to dissolve the brown sugar. Keep aside one cup brine to use in cooking chicken and pour the rest in a Ziploc bag.

2. Put the chicken in the bag and seal it for overnight marinating.

3. Remove chicken from brine and put in slow cooker. Add the reserved brine in the chicken and then add the liquid smoke. Cook by covering on low for 4 hours.

4. Remove the chicken and allow slight cooling after discarding the cooking juices.

5. Shred the chicken and return the pieces to the cooker to blend with barbecue sauce and then heat them thoroughly.

6. Serve by placing in the buns.

**Nutritional information:**

- Fat: 8 grams

- Carbohydrate: 43 grams

- Protein: 30 grams

## *BRAT SANDWICH*

- Yield: 10

- Time taken: 7 hours 15 minutes

**Ingredients:**

✓ 3 bottles of non-alcoholic beer

✓ 10 bratwurst links (uncooked)

- ✓ ¾ cup mayonnaise

- ✓ 1 large sweet onion (sliced)

- ✓ 2 tsp sweet pickle relish

- ✓ ¼ cup chili sauce

- ✓ 14 oz. sauerkraut (rinsed and drained)

- ✓ 1 tbsp. finely chopped onion

- ✓ 1/8 tsp pepper

- ✓ 10 hoagie buns (sliced)

- ✓ 2 cloves of garlic (minced)

- ✓ 2 tbsps. ketchup

- ✓ 10 slices of Swiss cheese

**Directions:**

1. In a skillet, cook the brats till they become brown and then drain off the excess fat.

2. Mix the beer with sliced onion, cooked brats and sauerkraut and put the mixture in a crock pot.

3. Cover the cooker and cook for 7 hours on low setting.

4. Keep the oven ready by preheating it at 350 degrees.

5. Mix mayonnaise with chili sauce, chopped onion, relish, ketchup, pepper and garlic in a bowl and spread the mixture over the sliced buns and top with cheese slice and cooked along with the sauerkraut.

6. Place the bread slices on a baking sheet and bake for 10 minutes, until the cheese melts. Serve

## SANDWICH WITH FRENCH STYLE DIP

- • Yield: 8

- Time taken: 8 hours 15 minutes

**Ingredients:**

- ✓ 1 tsp dried thyme
- ✓ 3 lb. beef rump roast
- ✓ 1½ tsp beef base
- ✓ 1 medium onion (cut into 4 pieces)
- ✓ ½ cup soy sauce
- ✓ 1 bay leaf
- ✓ 2 cloves of garlic (minced)
- ✓ 8 cups of water
- ✓ ½ tsp pepper
- ✓ 2 tbsps. Dijon mustard
- ✓ 8 slices of mozzarella cheese
- ✓ 2 lb. French bread
- ✓ 4½ oz. mushrooms 9drained and sliced)

**Directions:**

1. Mix the beef base with thyme and rum it all over the beef roast and place it in a crock pot.

2. Mix the onions with garlic, soy sauce, pepper and bay leaf in a bowl and pour the mixture over the beef in the cooker and then add water.

3. Cover the cooker and cook for about 8 hours on low setting ensuring the meat is tender.

4. Remove the meat to a cutting board and allow cooling.

5. Reserve the strained juices and onion separately and discard the bay leaf.

6. Slice the meat thinly and then assemble the sandwiches by slicing the bread into 16 equal pieces and spread the mustard all over the slices.

7. Place the cheese, beef, mushrooms and reserved onion and then place the top bread slices.

8. Serve the sandwiches with the reserved juices as the dip.

**Nutritional information**:

- Protein: 59 grams

- Fat: 19 grams

- Carbohydrates: 69 grams

# *ITALIAN TURKEY SANDWICHES*

- Yield: 12

- Time taken: 5 hours 15 minutes

**Ingredients:**

- ✓ 1 green pepper (chopped)

- ✓ 6 lb. turkey breast

- ✓ ¼ cup chili sauce

- ✓ 1 medium onion (chopped)

- ✓ 4 tsp beef Bouillon granules

- ✓ 3 tbsps. White vinegar

- ✓ 2 tbsps. Italian seasoning

- ✓ 12 hard rolls (split)

**Directions:**

1. Place turkey meat in a SLOW COOKER and add the pepper and onion pieces.

2. Mix the beef bouillon with chili sauce, seasoning mix and vinegar in a small bowl and pour the mixture over the meat in the cooker.

3. Cook by covering the cooker for 5 hours on low setting.

4. Allow cooling down and then shred the mat with two forks and return them to the cooker for heating up.

5. Prepare the sandwiches by placing a spoonful of meat mixture in between each roll of bread.

**Nutritional information:**

- Protein: 49 grams

- Fat: 4 grams

- Carbohydrates: 34 grams

# *DELIGHTFUL HAM SANDWICHES*

- Yield: 12

- Time taken: 4 hours 15 minutes

**Ingredients:**

- ✓ 2 cups of apple juice

- ✓ 3 lbs. ham (thinly sliced)

- ✓ ½ cup sweet pickle relish

- ✓ 1 tsp paprika

- ✓ 12 hard rolls (split)

✓ 2 tsp prepared mustard

✓ 2/3 cup packed brown sugar

**Directions:**

1. Separate the slices of ham and place them in the crock pot.

2. Mix the apple juice with brown sugar, mustard, paprika and relish in a small bowl and pour it over the ham.

3. Cover the cooker and cook on low setting for 4 hours.

4. Place a couple of ham slices in between the rolls and serve with some more sweet relish.

**Nutritional information:**

- Protein: 527grams

- Fat: 13 grams

- Carbohydrates: 52 grams

# *ITALIAN SAUSAGE SANDWICH*

- Yield: 10

- Time taken: 4 hours 15 minutes

**Ingredients:**

✓ 2 green peppers

✓ 48 oz. pasta sauce

✓ 2 onions (thinly sliced)

✓ ½ tsp crushed fennel seeds

✓ ½ tsp garlic powder

- ✓ 10 hoagie buns (split)

- ✓ 40 oz. Italian turkey sausage

**Directions:**

1. Mix the green peppers with pasta sauce, onions, garlic powder and fennel seeds in the crockpot and cook on low setting for 4 hours.

2. When the vegetables are almost ready, use the indoor grill to grill the sausage.

3. Place the sausage along with the cooked vegetables in between the buns and serve hot.

**Nutritional information:**

- Protein: 29 grams

- Fat: 15 grams

- Carbohydrates: 52 grams

# *SANDWICH WITH ROASTED BEEF*

- Yield: 15

- Time taken: 8 hours 15 minutes

**Ingredients:**

- ✓ 1 envelop of onion soup mix

- ✓ 4 lb. beef rump roast

- ✓ 6 oz. sliced mushrooms

- ✓ 2 celery rib (finely chopped)

- ✓ 1 can of condensed cream of mushroom soup

- ✓ 15 hard rolls (split)

## Directions:

1. Cut the roast into two large pieces and place it in the crock pot.

2. Mix the soup mixture along with the soup and celery in a bowl and pour it over the meat in the cooker and cook by covering it on low setting for 8 hours.

3. Just after 7 and half hours of cooking add the mushroom slices to the cooker and continue cooking for the remaining time.

4. Take out the meat from the cooker and allow a bit of cooling so that the meat can be easily shredded. Return them to the cooker for heating up again.

5. Place the meat with the juices and vegetable in between the rolls and serve.

## Nutritional information:

- Protein: 24 grams

- Fat: 8 grams

- Carbohydrates: 33 grams

# TASTY CHILI BEEF SANDWICH

- Yield: 8

- Time taken: 8 hours 15 minutes

## Ingredients:

- ✓ 1 envelop of chili seasoning

- ✓ 3 lbs. beef chuck roast

- ✓ 8 onion rolls (split)

- ✓ ½ cup BBQ sauce

✓ 8 slices of cheddar cheese

**Directions:**

1. Cut the roast into semi-small pieces and place them in the crock pot. Sprinkle the chili seasoning over the meat and pour the BBQ sauce on-top.

2. Cover the cooker and cook for 8 hours on low setting.

3. Remove the roast from the cooker and allow a bit of cooling so that the meat can be shredded easily.

4. Now return the shreds to the cooker to heat them up.

5. Arrange the cheese slices in the onion rolls and then place the cooked beef shreds and cover with the other half of the bun.

6. Serve hot.

**Nutritional information:**

- Protein: 47 grams

- Fat: 29 grams

- Carbohydrate: 29 grams

## SANDWICH WITH CHEESESTEAKS

- Yield: 6

- Time taken: 6 hours 15 minutes

**Ingredients:**

✓ 1½ lbs. beef top sirloin steak

✓ 2 onions (halved and sliced)

✓ 6 hoagie buns (split)

- ✓ 2 sweet red or green peppers

- ✓ 1 envelop onion soup mix

- ✓ 14 oz. beef broth

- ✓ 12 slices of provolone cheese (halved)

- ✓ Pickled hot cherry peppers

## Directions:

1. Put in the onions and peppers in the crockpot and add the beef along with soup mix and beef broth. Cover the pot and cook on low setting for 6 hours.

2. Place the buns on a baking sheet and place the meat mixture on the bottom of the buns and top with cheese.

3. Broil the sandwiches for 6 minutes until the cheese melts.

4. Serve with cherry peppers.

## Nutritional information:

- Protein: 44 grams

- Fat: 21 grams

- Carbohydrate: 45 grams

# HOT & SWEET PORK SANDWICH

- Yield: 10

- Total time: 8 hours 15 minutes

## Ingredients:

- ✓ 2 tbsps. Brown sugar

- ✓ 2 medium onions (sliced)

- ✓ ½ tsp pepper
- ✓ 1 tbsp. smoked paprika
- ✓ 5 lbs. boneless pork shoulder
- ✓ 1½ tsp salt
- ✓ ¼ cup cider vinegar
- ✓ ½ cup chicken broth
- ✓ 3 tbsps. Worcestershire sauce
- ✓ 3 tbsps. Soy sauce
- ✓ 1 tbsp. molasses
- ✓ 2 tbsps. Asian hot chili sauce
- ✓ 2 cloves of garlic, minced
- ✓ 3 cups of coleslaw mix
- ✓ 3 tbsps. Lime juice
- ✓ 2 tsp Dijon mustard
- ✓ 10 onion rolls (split)

**Directions:**

1. Put the sliced onions in the crock pot.

2. Mix the brown sugar with salt, paprika and pepper in a bowl and rub the mixture all over the roast and place the meat over the onions in the crock pot.

3. In a small bowl, mix the broth with soy sauce, vinegar, Worcestershire sauce, molasses, chili sauce, mustard and garlic and pour the mixture over the roast.

4. Cover the cooker and cook on low setting for 8 hours until the meat is tender.

5. Remove the meat and shred it using two forks. Skim out the fat from the cooking juices and preserve the juice.

6. Return the shredded meat to the cooker to make it hot.

7. Prepare the sandwiches by layering required amount of meat and cover with the top slice.

8. Mix the coleslaw with lime juice and serve it with the sandwich.

## *EASY TO MAKE BEEF STEAK SANDWICH*

- Yield: 8

- Time taken: 7 hours 15 minutes

**Ingredients:**

- ✓ ¼ cup soy sauce

- ✓ 2 lbs. boneless beef chuck steak

- ✓ 1 tsp ground ginger

- ✓ 1 tbsp. brown sugar

- ✓ 8 French rolls (split)

- ✓ 1 clove of garlic, minced

- ✓ 4 tsp cornstarch

- ✓ 2 tbsps. Water

- ✓ Rings of pineapple

- ✓ ¼ cup melted butter

- ✓ Chopped green onions

**Directions:**

1. Cut the beef steak into bite sized pieces and then put in the crock pot.

2. Mix the soy sauce with brown sugar, garlic and ginger and pour it over the steak pieces in the crock pot.

3. Cook by covering the SLOW COOKER for 7 hours and then remove the meat from the cooker.

4. Skim out the fat from the cooking juice and add water to it to increase the volume.

5. Pour the diluted juice in a saucepan and add the cornstarch and make a smooth paste.

6. Cook till it becomes bubbly and thick and then add the meat to it and hat up thoroughly.

7. Bush the rolls with melted butter and then broil for 5 minutes to make them lightly roasted.

8. Layer the sandwich with slices of onion and pineapple along with the cooked beef and serve.

**Nutritional information:**

- Protein: 29 grams

- Fat: 19 grams

- Carbohydrate: 33 grams

# *SLOW COOK TURKEY MEAT*

- Yield: 8

- Time taken: 4 hours 15 minutes

**Ingredients:**

- ✓ 1 small onion, chopped

- ✓ 1 lb. lean ground turkey

- ✓ ¼ cup green pepper, chopped

- ✓ ½ cup chopped celery

- ✓ ½ cup ketchup

- ✓ 10 oz. condensed tomato soup (undiluted)

- ✓ 2 tbsps. Prepared mustard

- ✓ 8 hamburger buns, split

- ✓ ¼ tsp pepper

- ✓ 1 tbsp. brown sugar

**Directions:**

1. In a large skillet, cook the turkey with cooking spray along with onions, celery and pepper until the meat is no longer pink in color.

2. Discard the excess juices and mix the tomato soup along with mustard, ketchup, pepper and brown sugar.

3. Pour the entire mixture into the crock pot, cover and for 4 hours on low setting.

4. Put the meat in between the bun and serve.

**Nutritional information:**

- Protein: 14 grams

- Fat: 7 grams

- Carbohydrate: 32 grams

# *BRISKET SANDWICH FANTASY*

- Yield: 12

- Time taken: 8 hours 15 minutes

**Ingredients:**

- ✓ 2 tbsps. cider vinegar
- ✓ 5 lbs. beef brisket
- ✓ 1½ cup water
- ✓ ½ cup Worcestershire sauce
- ✓ 2 cloves of garlic, minced
- ✓ 1½ tsp chili powder
- ✓ 1½ tsp beef bouillon granules
- ✓ ½ tsp cayenne pepper
- ✓ 2 tbsps. Butter
- ✓ 1 tsp ground mustard
- ✓ ¼ tsp garlic salt
- ✓ ½ tsp hot pepper sauce
- ✓ 2 tbsps. Brown sugar
- ✓ ½ cup ketchup
- ✓ 12 onion rolls

**Directions:**

1. Cut the beef brisket into half and then place it in the crockpot.

2. In a small bowl, mix water with Worcestershire sauce, garlic, vinegar, beef bouillon, chili powder, mustard, garlic salt and cayenne.

3. Reserve half cup of this mixture in the fridge and pour the rest over the beef.

4. Cover and cook for 8 hours on low setting until the meat is tender.

5. Take out the meat from the SLOW COOKER without its cooking juices and skim out the fat from the liquid.

6. Shred the meat with fork and then return the shredded pieces to the crockpot.

7. In a saucepan, mix the ketchup, brown sugar, pepper sauce, butter and reserved mixture from the fridge, boil then simmer for some time.

8. Place the shredded beef on the buns and drizzle with this sauce to serve.

**Nutritional information:**

- Protein: 37 grams

- Fat: 11 grams

- Carbohydrate: 38 grams

# SLOW COOK PORK RECIPES

## *BARBERCUE PORK RIBS*

- 15 min

- Total Time: 10 hr.

- Servings: 4

**Ingredients:**

- ✓ 3 1/2 lb. pork loin back ribs

- ✓ 4 tbsp. packed brown sugar

- ✓ 1 tsp salt

- ✓ 1/2 tsp pepper

- ✓ 3 tbsp. liquid smoke
- ✓ 2 chopped garlic cloves
- ✓ 1 sliced onion (medium)
- ✓ 8 tbsp. cola
- ✓ 1 1/2 cups barbecue sauce

Directions:

1. The following ingredients will be mixed: liquid smoke, pepper, sugar and salt.

2. The ribs will be rubbed in this newly obtained mixture.

3. Transfer the ribs in a greased slow cooker (4-5 quart) and pour cola over them.

4. After covering the slow cooker, set the heat on Low and cook for about 9 hours.

5. Make sure the ribs are tender before ending the cooking process. After removing the ribs from the slow cooker, drain and remove the liquid.

6. The barbecue sauce will be poured a bowl. After dipping the ribs in the barbecue sauce, place them again in the slow cooker.

7. The rest of barbecue sauce will also be poured on over the ribs, in the slow cooker.

8. After covering the slow cooker, set the heat on Low and cook for another 60 minutes.

**Nutrition Information:**

- Calories: 890

- Total Fat: 60 g

- Cholesterol: 230 mg

- Sodium: 1540 mg

- Total Carbohydrate: 32 g

- Protein: 58 g

# *DELICIOUS MEXICAN SANDWICHES*

- Prep Time: 15 min

- Total Time: 10 hr.

- Servings: 18

**Ingredients:**

- ✓ 2 ½ lb. pork loin roast

- ✓ 1 thinly sliced onion (medium size)

- ✓ 2 cups barbecue sauce

- ✓ 12 tbsp. salsa

- ✓ 1 tbsp. chili powder

- ✓ 1 tsp ground cumin

- ✓ 1 lb. stir-fry bell peppers and onions (frozen)

- ✓ 1/2 tsp salt

- ✓ 18 flour tortillas

- ✓ Cheese (shredded; optional)

- ✓ Guacamole (optional)

- ✓ Sour cream (optional)

**Directions:**

6. The meat will be transferred in a slow cooker. Top with onion.

7. Mix the salsa with the following ingredients: cumin, barbecue sauce and chili powder.

8. Top the onion with this newly obtained mixture.

9. After covering the slow cooker, set the heat on Low and cook for 9-10 hours.

10. After removing transferring the meat on a cutting board, shredded it with 2 forks.

11. The meat will now be returned to the slow cooker and mixed well with the rest of ingredients. Add salt and stir-fry vegetables.

12. Mix well. Again, cover the slow cooker. Set the heat on High and cook for half an hour. Make sure the vegetables are tender before ending the cooking process.

13. Each tortilla will be filled with 8 tbsp. pork mixture. The end of tortilla will be folded up 1 inch over the filling.

14. The right and the left sides of the tortilla will be folded over the folded end, overlapping. The remaining end will be folded down.

15. You can serve the Pork Fajitas with sour cream/ cheese/ guacamole.

**Nutrition Information:**

- Calories: 290
- Total Fat: 8 g
- Cholesterol: 40 mg
- Sodium: 620 mg
- Total Carbohydrate: 37 g
- Protein: 18 g

# *PORK CHOPS FRUITS COMBO*

- Prep Time: 15 min
- Total Time: 8 hr.
- Servings: 6

**Ingredients:**

- ✓ 6 ounces stuffing turkey flavor
- ✓ 2 chopped celery stalks (medium size)
- ✓ 1 tart cooking apple
- ✓ 1 chopped onion (medium size)
- ✓ 1 cup cherries (dried)
- ✓ 4 tbsp. melted butter
- ✓ 16 tbsp. chicken broth
- ✓ 6 pork loin chops

**Directions:**

1. All the ingredients will be mixed, ½ of the mixture will be transferred in a greased slow cooker (4-5 quart).

2. Place the pork chops over the mixture, inside the slow cooker, and add the remaining mixture over the pork chops, too.

3. After covering the slow cooker, set the heat on Low and cook for 7-8 hours.

4. Make sure the pork chops are tender before ending the cooking progress.

**Nutrition Information:**

- Calories: 485

- Total Fat: 17 g

- Cholesterol: 85 mg

- Sodium: 870 mg

- Total Carbohydrate: 58 g

- Protein: 29 g

# GRILLED PORK RIBS

- Prep Time: 30 min

- Total Time: 9 hr.

- Servings: 6

## Ingredients:

- ✓ 3 1/2 lb. pork loin back ribs
- ✓ 4 tbsp. packed brown sugar
- ✓ 1 tsp salt
- ✓ 1/2 tsp pepper
- ✓ 3 tbsp. liquid smoke
- ✓ 2 finely chopped cloves garlic
- ✓ 1 sliced onion (medium size)
- ✓ 8 tbsp. cola
- ✓ 1 1/2 cups barbecue sauce

## Directions:

1. Mix the following ingredients: liquid smoke, sugar, garlic and pepper. This mixture will be rubbed into the ribs.

2. Split each rib into 4 pieces and layer the pieces and the onion in a greased slow cooker (4-5 quart). Add cola over these pieces.

3. After covering the slow cooker, set the heat on Low and cook for 8-9 hours. Make sure the ribs are tender before ending the cooking process.

4. The ribs will be removed from the slow cooker. Drain and discard the liquid from the slow cooker.

5. The ribs will be transferred on a grill (gas or coal). After spreading the barbecue sauce on the ribs, cover and grill for a quarter of an hour over medium heat (4-6 inches from the heat).

## Nutrition Information:

- Calories: 590

- Total Fat: 40g

- Cholesterol: 155mg

- Sodium: 1030mg

- Total Carbohydrate: 21g

# *ISLAND STYLE PORK RIBS*

- Prep Time: 15 min

- Total Time: 8 hr.

- Servings: 6

**Ingredients:**

- ✓ Slow Cooker Liners

- ✓ Ribs

    - ✓ 2 pounds country-style pork loin ribs (bones will be removed)

    - ✓ 1 finely chopped clove garlic

    - ✓ 1 sliced onion (small size)

    - ✓ 8 ounces pineapple in juice (crushed and undrained)

## Sauce

- ✓ 12 tbsp. ketchup

- ✓ 3 tbsp. packed brown sugar

- ✓ 3 tbsp. hoisin sauce

- ✓ 1 tsp grated gingerroot

- ✓ Hot cooked rice (optional ingredient)

Directions:

1. The bottom and the sides of the slow cooker (5-6 ½ quart) will be lined using the liners that are mentioned in the ingredients list.

2. The pork ribs, the garlic and the onion will be transferred in the slow cooker. ½ of the pineapple and a part of the juice will be spooned over the pork ribs.

3. The rest of the pineapple and the remaining juice will be reserved.

4. After covering the slow cooker, set the heat on Low and cook for 9-10 hours.

5. Drain and remove cooking juices from the slow cooker half an hour before serving the pork ribs.

6. Don't forget to wipe the edge of the cooker clean.

7. Mix the following ingredients in a different bowl: hoisin sauce, ketchup, pineapple and juice, gingerroot and sugar.

8. Spoon the newly obtained mixture over the pork ribs.

9. Cover the slow cooker, set the heat on High and cook for about half an hour. Make sure the ribs are glazed before stopping the cooking process.

10. The pork ribs can be served with rice.

**Nutrition Information:**

- Calories: 390

- Trans Fat: 0g

- Cholesterol: 90mg

- Sodium: 530mg

- Total Carbohydrate: 25g

- Sugars: 20g

- Protein: 22g

## TEX-MEX FAJITAS RECIPE

- Prep Time: 20 min

- Total Time: 8 hr.

- Servings: 16

**Ingredients:**

✓ Liners for the slow cooker

- ✓ 2 ½ lb. pork loin roast (the bones and the excess fat will be removed)

- ✓ 2 tbsp. fajita seasoning

- ✓ 16 tbsp. salsa (thick and chunky)

- ✓ 1 pound frozen stir-fry bell peppers and onions (thawed)

- ✓ 16 flour tortillas for burritos (the tortillas will be warmed)

- ✓ 8 ounces taco cheese (shredded)

- ✓ 16 tbsp. sour cream (optional)

Directions:

6. The liners will be placed on the bottom and on the sides of the slow cooker. The top of the liner will also cover the rim of the slow cooker.

7. The meat will be transferred in the slow cooker and the fajita seasoning will be spread over it. Salsa will be used for topping the meat.

8. After covering the slow cooker, set the heat on Low and cook for 9-10 hours.

9. The pork meat will be transferred on a cutting board and it will be shredded with 2 forks. Then, the meat will be placed in the slow cooker, again.

10. After mixing thoroughly the meat, the fry-vegetables will be stirred in. The slow cooker will be covered and the heat will be set on High.

11. The cooking process will be continued for another half an hour. Make sure the vegetables are tender before ending the cooking process.

12. 8 tbsp. meat mixture will be spooned on each tortilla. Add cheese, as well. The Fajitas can be served with sour cream, too.

**Nutrition Information:**

- Calories: 320

- Total Fat: 14g

- Cholesterol: 60mg

- Sodium: 730mg

- Total Carbohydrate: 24g

- Sugars: 2g

- Protein: 22g

## *CHEESY PORK CHOPS WITH TOMATO SAUCE*

- Prep Time: 10 min

- Total Time: 4 hr.

- Servings: 6

**Ingredients:**

- ✓ 6 pork loin chops

- ✓ 1/2 tsp salt

- ✓ 1/4 tsp pepper

- ✓ 1 tbsp. vegetable oil

✓ 1 chopped onion (medium size)

✓ 2 cups tomato pasta sauce

✓ 4 cups cooked orzo

✓ 4 ounces mozzarella cheese (shredded)

## Directions:

1. Heat the oil in a skillet (12-inch), over medium high-heat. The pork chops will be sprinkled with salt and pepper.

2. Transfer the pork chops in the skillet, too, and cook them for 5 minutes. Turn the pork chops once during this cooking process.

3. Transfer the pork chops in a slow cooker (3 ½ - 4 quart) and sprinkle onion over them. Transfer pasta sauce in the slow cooker, as well.

4. After covering the slow cooker, set the heat on Low and cook for 5-6 hours.

5. Orzo will be placed on the platter. Transfer the pork chops and the sauce on the platter, too, over orzo.

6. Spread the cheese over the pork chops, too.

## Nutrition Information:

- Calories: 510

- Total Fat: 19g

- Cholesterol: 85mg

- Sodium: 880mg

- Total Carbohydrate: 46g

- Sugars: 9g

- Protein: 38g

## *PULLED PORK*

- Prep Time: 10 min

- Total Time: 6 hr.

- Servings: 4

### Ingredients:

- 1 tbsp. kosher (coarse) salt

- 1 tbsp. paprika

- 1 tsp garlic powder

- 1 tsp packed brown sugar

- 1 pork loin roast (2.5-3 pounds)

- 1 cup water

- 1 cup barbecue sauce

### Directions:

1. Mix the following ingredients: paprika, sugar, and salt and garlic powder.

2. The pork roast will be rinsed (use cool water). The pork chops will be rubbed in the above mentioned mixture

3. Transfer the pork chops in a greased slow cooker (4-6 quart) and add water to side of meat.

4. Cover the slow cooker, set the heat on High and cook for 5-6 hours.

5. The meat will be shredded with 2 forks inside the slow cooker. The barbecue sauce will be stirred in, too.

**Nutrition Information:**

- Calories: 510

# SLOW COOKER STEW RECIPES

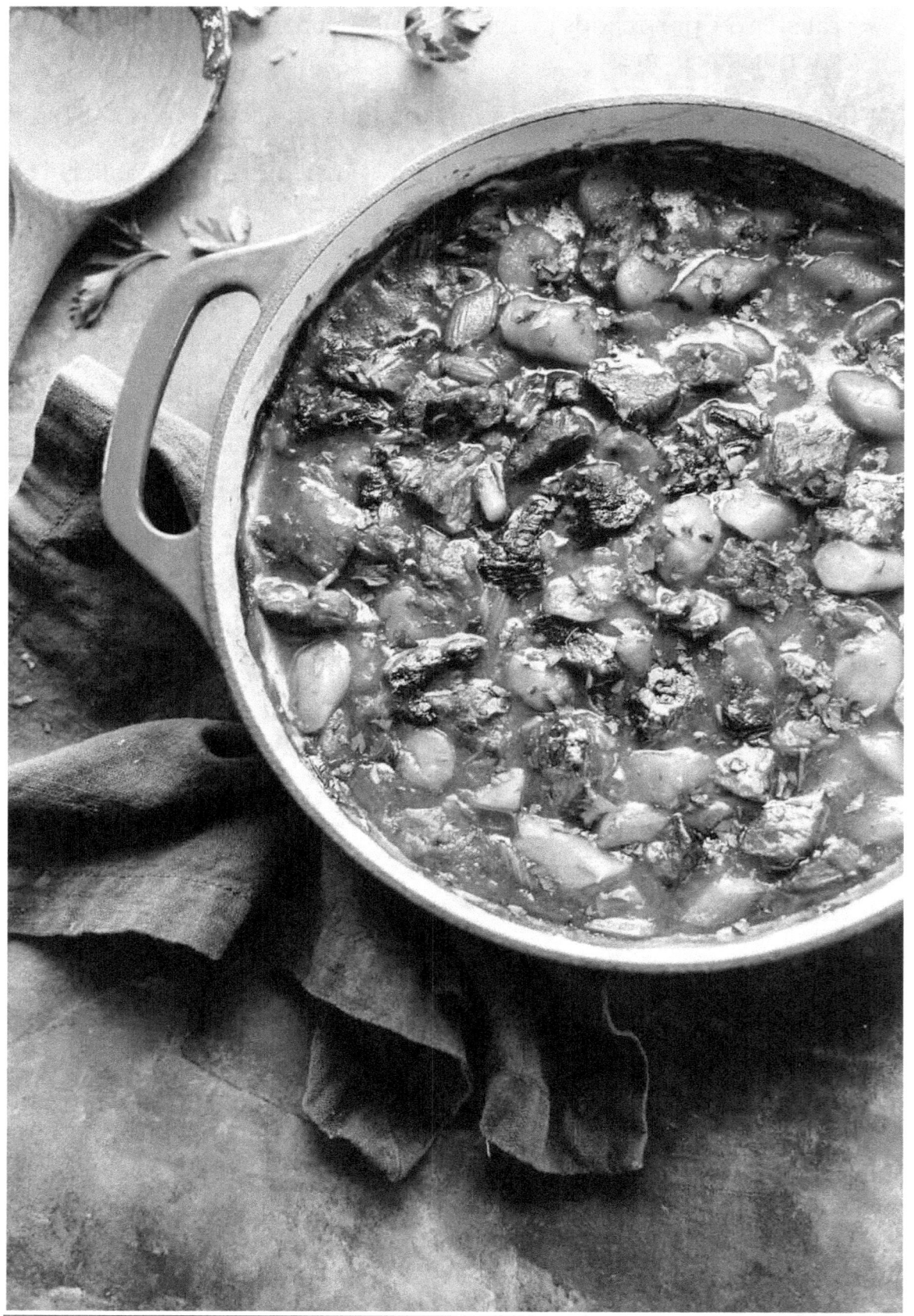

# CHICKEN MARSALA SOUP

- Prep Time: 10 min
- Total Time: 5 hr.
- Servings: 8

**Ingredients:**

- ✓ 2 finely chopped cloves garlic
- ✓ 1 tbsp. vegetable oil
- ✓ 8 chicken breasts (bones and skin will be removed
- ✓ 1/2 tsp salt
- ✓ 1/2 tsp pepper
- ✓ 6 ounces mushrooms (sliced and drained)
- ✓ 16 tbsp. sweet Marsala wine (this ingredient can be replaced with chicken broth)
- ✓ 8 tbsp. water
- ✓ 4 tbsp. cornstarch
- ✓ 3 tbsp. fresh parsley (chopped)

**Directions:**

1. Place the oil and the garlic in a greased slow cooker (4-5 quart). After spreading the salt and the pepper over the chicken, transfer it in the slow cooker.

2. Add mushrooms over the chicken breast and pour wine.

3. After covering the slow cooker, set the heat on Low and cook for 5-6 hours.

4. Transfer the chicken from slow cooker to a plate and keep it warm by covering the chicken. Using a different bowl, mix cornstarch with water.

5. Stop mixing when the mixture is smooth. Stir the newly obtained mixture into the slow cooker. Set the heat on High and cook for 10 minutes.

6. Make sure the sauce is thick enough before ending the cooking process. Place the chicken back in the slow cooker.

7. The mushroom mixture will be spooned over the chicken breast and parsley will be sprinkled over the mixture, as well.

**Nutrition Information:**

- Calories: 440

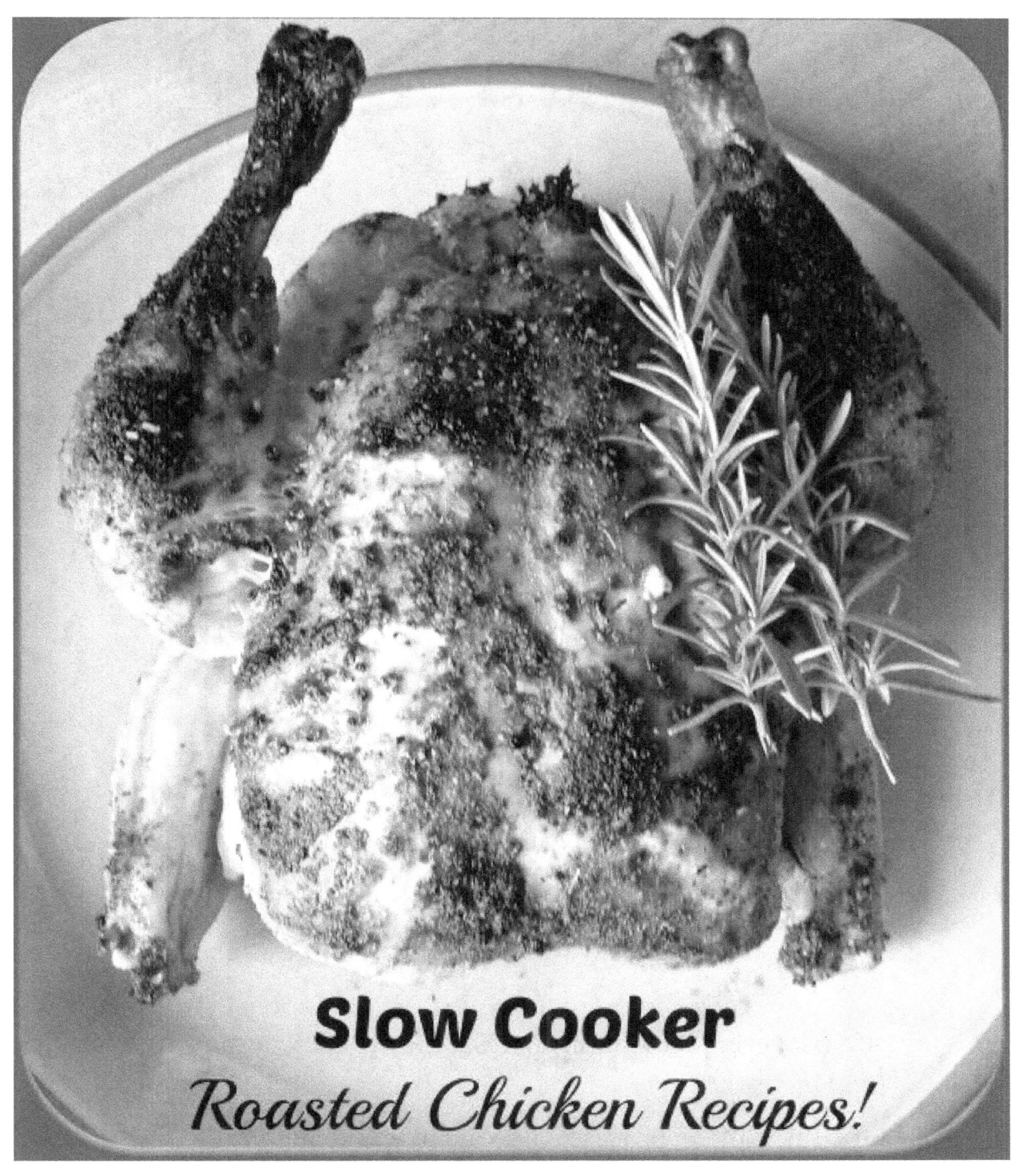

**Slow Cooker**

*Roasted Chicken Recipes!*

## TEXAS STEW SLOW COOK

- Prep Time: 10 min

- Total Time: 8 hr.

- Servings: 6

## Ingredients:

- ✓ 1 1/4 lb. beef stew meat

- ✓ 4 potatoes (unpeeled, cut into 1-inch pieces)

- ✓ 8 tbsp. onion (chopped)

- ✓ 1 tsp salt

- ✓ 1/4 tsp pepper

- ✓ 28 oz. beans in barbecue sauce (baked)

## Directions:

1. The following ingredients will be mixed in a slow cooker (3 ½-4 quart): potatoes, salt and pepper, beef and onion.

2. The baked beans will also be spread over the above mentioned mixture.

3. After covering the slow cooker, set the heat on Low and cook for 9-10 hours.

4. Stop the cooking process when the beef is tender.

## Nutrition Information:

- Calories: 370

- Total Fat: 12g

- Cholesterol: 65mg

- Sodium: 1030mg

- Total Carbohydrate: 46g

- Protein: 28g

# *ITALIAN TURKEY SOUP*

- Prep Time: 30 min

- Total Time: 9 hr.

- Servings: 6

## Ingredients:

- ✓ Slow Cooker Liners

- ✓ 6 cups water

- ✓ 16 ounces navy beans, (dried; sorted and rinsed)

- ✓ 3 cups chicken broth

- ✓ 4 tbsp. olive oil

- ✓ 12 tbsp. parsley (chopped)

- ✓ 1 tbsp. Italian seasoning

- ✓ 2 tbsp. garlic (chopped)

- ✓ 1 1/2 tsp salt

- ✓ 1/2 tsp pepper

- ✓ 1.5-2.25 lb. turkey thighs (the skin will be removed)

- ✓ 1 1/2 cups frozen green beans (cut, thawed)

**Directions:**

1. The liners will be placed in a slow cooker bowl (5-6 ½ quart). The liners will fit the sides and the bottom of the slow cooker bowl.

2. Furthermore, the top of the liner should cover the rim of the bowl, as well.

3. The water will be brought to a boil in a saucepan (3-quart) over medium-high heat. Transfer the navy beans inside the slow cooker. Simmer for about 10 minutes over medium-low heat (do not cover the saucepan).

4. Drain and, using cold water, rinse. Transfer the navy beans in the slow cooker and add broth, as well.

5. In a different bowl, mix the Italian seasoning with 8 tbsp. parsley, half tsp salt and pepper, olive oil and garlic.

6. The mixture will be spread (and pressed) over the thighs. Transfer them in the slow cooker, over beans. After covering the slow cooker, set the heat on Low and cook for 8-9 hours.

7. Make sure the beans are tender and the meat can be pulled apart easily when using a fork, before ending the cooking process.

8. After removing the thighs from the slow cooker, set the heat on high, add remaining 1 tsp salt and green beans in the slow cooker, too, cover and cook for 15-20 minutes.

9. Top the cooking process when the vegetables are hot. During this cooking process remove the bones from the thighs.

10. Before serving, transfer the bean mixture in shallow bowls. Add turkey and spread the remaining parsley over it.

**Nutrition Information:**

- Calories: 480

- Total Fat: 14g

- Cholesterol: 90mg

- Sodium: 1080mg

- Total Carbohydrate: 49g

- Sugars: 2g

- Protein: 39g

## *TUSCAN BEEF STEW*

- Prep Time: 15 min

- Total Time: 12 hr.

- Servings: 6

**Ingredients:**

- ✓ 1 lb. beef stew meat

- ✓ 1 tsp beef base

- ✓ 3 carrots (large size; cut them into 1-inch pieces)
- ✓ 2 stalks celery (medium size; cut into 1-inch pieces)
- ✓ 2 finely chopped cloves garlic
- ✓ 1 coarsely chopped onion (medium size)
- ✓ 1/4 tsp pepper
- ✓ 19 oz. cannellini (white kidney) beans (rinsed and drained)
- ✓ 28 oz. crushed tomatoes in puree (undrained)
- ✓ 12 oz. beef gravy
- ✓ 2 tsp Italian seasoning
- ✓ 1 tsp sugar
- ✓ 2 cups frozen green beans (cut)

## Directions:

1. Set aside the following ingredients: sugar, Italian seasoning and frozen green beans.

2. The rest of the ingredients will be transferred in a slow cooker (3 ½-4 quart).

3. After covering the slow cooker, set the heat on Low and cook for 11-12 hours.

4. Stir in the remaining ingredients (which have been set aside at Step 1). Cover the slow cooker again, set the heat on High and cook for another quarter of an hour.

5. Stop cooking process when the vegetables are tender.

## Nutrition Information:

- Calories: 340

- Total Fat: 11g

- Cholesterol: 50mg

- Sodium: 800mg

- Total Carbohydrate: 41g

- Protein: 29g

## *FABULOUS BEEF STEW*

- Prep Time: 35 min

- Total Time: 8 hr.

- Servings: 6

**Ingredients:**

- ✓ Slow Cooker Liners

- ✓ 2 tbsp. butter (margarine can be used, as well)

- ✓ 1 1/2 onions sweet onions (halved and thinly sliced)

- ✓ 2 tsp sugar

- ✓ 2 tsp thyme leaves (fresh ; chopped)

- ✓ 1 1/2 pound beef stew

- ✓ 1 cup broth (beef flavored)

- ✓ 0.8-1 oz. onion gravy mix

- ✓ 2 cups carrots (diagonally cut 1-inch pieces)

✓ 1 cup parsnips (diagonally cut 1-inch pieces)

✓ 8 tbsp. sweet peas (frozen)

Directions:

1. The liners will be placed in a slow cooker bowl (5-6 ½ quart). The liners will fit the sides and the bottom of the slow cooker bowl.

2. Furthermore, the top of the liner should cover the rim of the bowl, as well.

3. The butter will be melted over medium-low heat in a skillet (10-inch). Add onions and sugar and cook for about half an hour.

4. Stir constantly and stop the cooking process when the onions become deep golden brown (caramelized).

5. Add the stew meat and thyme, as well. Stir. Transfer the mixture in the slow cooker.

6. Mix the following ingredients in a different bowl: gravy mix and beef flavored broth.

7. This newly obtained mixture will be poured in the slow cooker, over the beef mixture. Add carrots and parsnips over the mixture, as well.

8. After covering the slow cooker, set the heat on Low and cook for 8-9 hours.

9. Make sure the meat and the vegetables are tender before ending the cooking process.

10. Add peas and stir. Cover the slow cooker again and cook for another 10-15 minutes.

## Nutrition Information:

- Calories: 290

- Total Fat: 15g

- Cholesterol: 60mg

- Sodium: 450mg

- Total Carbohydrate: 21g

- Sugars: 9g

- Protein: 18g

## *BURGUNDY STEW*

- Prep Time: 25 min

- Total Time: 9 hr.

- Servings: 8

**Ingredients:**

**Stew**

- ✓ 2 pounds beef bottom or top round (bones, if any, will be removed; cut the beef into 1-inch pieces)

- ✓ 4 carrots (medium size; cut the carrots into 1/4-inch slices)

- ✓ 2 sliced stalks celery (medium size)

- ✓ 2 sliced onions (medium onion)

- ✓ 14.5-15 ounces tomatoes (diced and undrained)

- ✓ 9-10 ounces mushrooms (sliced and drained)

- ✓ 12 tbsp. dry red wine (beef flavored broth can be used as a replacement)

- ✓ 1 1/2 tsp salt

- ✓ 1 tsp thyme leaves (dried)

- ✓ 1 tsp ground mustard

- ✓ 1/4 tsp pepper

- ✓ 14 tbsp. water

- ✓ 3 tbsp. all-purpose flour

**Dumplings:**

- ✓ 1 ½ cups bisques mix

- ✓ ½ tsp thyme leaves (dried)

- ✓ ¼ tsp sage leaves (dried, crushed)

- ✓ 8 tbsp. milk

**Directions:**

1. Set the flour and the water aside. Mix all the stew the ingredients in a slow cooker (4-5 quart).

2. After covering the slow cooker, set the heat on Low and cook for 9-10 hours.

3. If you will be using the High heat setting, cook for just 4-5 hours.

4. Flour and water will be mixed in a bowl. Add the meat mixture progressively and stir.

5. Mix half tsp thyme, bisques mix and dried sage leaves in a different bowl.

6. Add milk and stir until the bisques mix is moistened. Spoonful of dough will be dropped onto the meat mixture.

7. After covering the slow cooker again, set the heat on High and cook for another 30-35 minutes.

8. Stop the cooking process when an inserted toothpick comes out clean.

**Nutrition Information:**

- Calories: 300

- Total Fat: 7g

- Cholesterol: 65mg

- Sodium: 990mg

- Total Carbohydrate: 28g

- Sugars: 6g

- Protein: 30g

# *BEIJING PORK STEW*

- Prep Time: 25 min

- Total Time: 7 hr.

- Servings: 8

**Ingredients:**

- ✓ 2 pounds country-style pork ribs (bones will be removed; cut into 2-inch pieces)

- ✓ 3 carrots (medium size; cut into 1-inch slices)
- ✓ 2 onions (medium size; cut into 1-inch wedges)
- ✓ 8 ounces whole mushrooms (fresh; cut in half if they are too large)
- ✓ 8 ounces whole water chestnuts (drained)
- ✓ 8 ounces bamboo shoots (drained)
- ✓ 12 tbsp. hoisin sauce
- ✓ 5 tbsp. soy sauce (reduced-sodium)
- ✓ 4 finely chopped cloves garlic (large size)
- ✓ 1 tbsp. finely chopped gingerroot
- ✓ 4 cups water
- ✓ 2 cups long-grain white rice (uncooked)
- ✓ 2 tbsp. cornstarch
- ✓ 3 tbsp. water
- ✓ 5 tbsp. coarsely chopped cilantro (lightly packed)

Directions:

1. The following ingredients will be layered in a greased slow cooker (5-6 quart): pork, onions, carrots, water chestnuts, mushrooms, bamboo shoots.

2. Stir together in a different bowl the following ingredients: soy sauce, gingerroot, 8 tbsp. hoisin sauce and garlic.

3. Pour this newly obtained mixture into slow cooker.

4. After covering the slow cooker, set the heat on Low and cook for 8-9 hours.

5. 60 minutes before the above mentioned cooking process will end, place in a skillet (3-quart) water and rice and bring them to a boil over high heat.

6. Set the heat on Low, cover the skillet and simmer for 15-20 minutes. Make sure the rice is tender and the water is absorbed.

7. The meat and the vegetables will be transferred from the slow cooker to a large bowl, using a slotted spoon.

8. The bowl will be covered (this is needed for keeping the pork and the vegetables warm). The fat (if any) will be removed the liquid in slow cooker.

9. Transfer the liquid into a saucepan (1-quart). The remaining 4 tbsp. of hoisin sauce will be stirred into the liquid.

10. Bring the liquid to a boil. 3 tbsp. of water will be mixed with cornstarch in a different bowl.

11. Stir this new mixture into liquid. Stir constantly and cook. Stop the cooking process when thickened. Pour over the above mentioned pork mixture and stir.

12. Cilantro will be spread over the stew.

13. Serve the stew over rice.


**Nutrition Information:**

- Calories: 510

- Total Fat: 15g

- Cholesterol: 70mg

- Sodium: 810mg

- Total Carbohydrate: 63g

- Sugars: 5g

- Protein: 30g

## *Spicy Beef Stew*

- Prep Time: 10 min

- Total Time: 9 hr.

- Servings: 6

**Ingredients:**

- ✓ 1 1/2 pounds beef stew meat

- ✓ 4 potatoes (medium size, cut into 1-inch pieces)

- ✓ 1 coarsely chopped onion (medium size)

- ✓ 43.5 ounces diced tomatoes with zesty mild green chilies (undrained)

- ✓ 1 3/4 cups broth (beef flavored)

- ✓ 1 tbsp. chili powder

- ✓ 2 tsp ground cumin

- ✓ 1 tsp garlic salt

- ✓ a dash of pepper

**Directions:**

1. All the ingredients will be mixed in a slow cooker (3 ½-4 quart).

2. After covering the slow cooker, set the heat on Low and cook for 9-10 hours.

## Nutrition Information:

- Calories: 390
- Total Fat: 14g
- Cholesterol: 65mg
- Sodium: 1130mg
- Total Carbohydrate: 37g
- Sugars: 11g
- Protein: 28g

## *SEOUL BEEF STEW*

- Prep Time: 10 min
- Total Time: 9 hr.
- Servings: 6

## Ingredients:

- ✓ 2 pounds beef stew meat (cut into 1-inch pieces)
- ✓ 16 ounces ready-to-eat baby-cut carrots
- ✓ 6 green onions (cut the onions into 1-inch pieces)
- ✓ 2 chopped cloves garlic

- ✓ 8 tbsp. tomato juice
- ✓ 4 tbsp. soy sauce
- ✓ 3 tbsp. sugar
- ✓ 2 tbsp. sesame oil (vegetable oil)
- ✓ 1/4 tsp pepper
- ✓ 2 tsp cornstarch
- ✓ 4 tsp cold water
- ✓ 3 cups cooked rice (hot)

**Directions:**

1. Mix the following ingredients in a greased slow cooker (3-4 quart): carrots, garlic, soy sauce, oil, beef, onions, tomato juice, sugar and pepper.

2. After covering the slow cooker, set the heat on Low and cook for 9-11 hours. If you will set the heat on High, reduce the cooking time to 5 – 5 ½ hours).

3. Mix water with cornstarch in a different bowl. Make sure they blend well. Stir into the mixture in the slow cooker.

4. Cover the slow cooker again, set the heat on High and cook for another 20 minutes.

5. Make sure the mixture is slightly thickened before ending the cooking process.

6. Serve this stew with rice.

**Nutrition Information:**

- Calories: 470

- Total Fat: 21g

- Cholesterol: 80mg

- Sodium: 1070mg

- Total Carbohydrate: 39g

- Sugars: 11g

- Protein: 31g

# SLOW COOKER TURKEY RECIPES

## *TURKEY TETRAZZINI*

- Prep Time: 15 min

- Total Time: 4 hr.

- Servings: 4

**Ingredients:**

- ✓ 10.5 ounces cream of chicken (this ingredient can be replaced with mushroom soup, too)

- ✓ 1 cup vegetable broth (this ingredient can be replaced with chicken broth, too)

- ✓ 8 tbsp. heavy cream

- ✓ 4 tbsp. white wine (dry)

- ✓ 2 cups diced turkey breast (cooked)

- ✓ 2 cups broken spaghetti noodles (uncooked)

- ✓ 1 cup peas (frozen)

- ✓ 1 cup shredded Parmesan cheese (divided)

- ✓ 4 tbsp. white onion (chopped)

- ✓ 2 tbsp. pimientos (chopped)

- ✓ 4.5 ounces mushrooms (sliced and drained)

- ✓ 1 tsp parsley (dried)

- ✓ 1/4 tsp paprika

- ✓ 1/2 tsp salt

- ✓ 1/2 tsp pepper

- ✓ Pinch nutmeg

- ✓ fresh parsley, for serving

**Directions:**

1. Stir together the following ingredients in a large bowl: broth, wine, soup and cream.

2. The following ingredients will be added, as well: noodles, 8 tbsp. cheese (Parmesan), pimientos, dried parsley, salt, nutmeg, turkey, peas, onion, mushrooms, paprika and pepper.

3. Stir and make sure all ingredients are well combined.

4. The above mentioned mixture will be transferred into a lightly greased slow cooker.

5. The remaining Parmesan cheese will be sprinkled over the top of the mixture in the slow cooker.

6. After covering the slow cooker, set the heat on Low and cook for 4-5 hours. Make sure the noodles are tender before ending the cooking process.

7. Fresh parsley will be used for topping the mixture. If needed, add some more salt and/ or pepper.

# TACO-SEASONED TURKEY

- Prep Time: 10 min

- Total Time: 2 hr.

- Servings: 6

## Ingredients:

- 1 ounce taco seasoning mix

- 4 tbsp. honey

- 2 tbsp. melted butter

- 1 turkey breast half

- 1 cup chicken broth

## Directions:

1. The taco seasoning mix and the honey will be stirred into the melted butter. Rub over and under the skin of turkey breast.

2. Transfer on foil-lined rimmed cookie-sheet. Place in the refrigerator and keep it there for at least 60 minutes (do not exceed 12 hours).

3. The chicken stock will be transferred into a slow cooker (5-6 quart). The turkey will be transferred in the slow cooker, as well.

4. After covering the slow cooker, set the heat on High and cook for 2 hours and a half.

5. If you will set the heat on Low, cook for 5 hours. In both situations, make sure the juice of turkey is clear when cutting the center (or the thickest part).

6. The turkey will be removed from the slow cooker and set aside for about 10 minutes (make sure it is covered with foil.

7. Slice turkey crosswise before serving.

# SAUSAGE BREAKFAST CASSEROLE

- Prep Time: 20 min

- Total Time: 3 hr.

- Servings: 8

**Ingredients:**

- ✓ 12 eggs

- ✓ 12 tbsp. evaporated low-fat 2% milk (canned)

- ✓ 1/2 tsp red pepper flakes (crushed)

- ✓ 1/2 tsp salt

- ✓ 1/4 tsp freshly ground black pepper

- ✓ 4 ounces sharp Cheddar cheese (shredded; reduced-fat)

- ✓ 8 tbsp. green onions (chopped)

- ✓ 1 cup Colby-Monterey Jack cheese (shredded; reduced-fat)

- ✓ -20 ounces shredded hash brown potatoes (refrigerated, cooked)

- ✓ 9.5-10 ounces turkey sausage crumbles (refrigerated, cooked)

- ✓ 8 tbsp. roasted red bell peppers (chopped)

**Directions:**

1. Fold foil into thirds and line the sides of a slow cooker (5-quart). Grease the slow cooker with cooking spray.

2. The eggs will be beaten with a whisk, in a bowl, together with the milk, the pepper, the salt and the pepper flakes.

3. Refrigerate 12 tbsp. Cheddar cheese and 2 tbsp. green onions while the breakfast casserole cooks.

4. The remaining cheeses will be stirred together in a different bowl.

5. Layer half in the slow cooker each of the potatoes, roasted peppers, sausage, green onions (the remaining quantity) and cheese.

6. This layering will be repeated. Egg mixture will be poured over these layers, too.

7. After covering the slow cooker, set the heat on Low and cook for 4-5 hours.

8. Make sure the temperature has reached 160 degrees F/ 70 degrees C in center before ending this cooking process. Furthermore, the mixture must be set.

9. After turning off the slow cooker, the reserved cheese and green onions will be spread over the top of the casserole.

10. Cover the slow cooker and wait 10 minutes for the cheese to melt.

11. The foil will be removed before serving (use a table knife to loosen the edges).

**Nutrition Information:**

- Calories: 400

- Total Fat: 18g

- Cholesterol: 330mg

- Sodium: 710mg

- Total Carbohydrate: 29g

- Sugars: 5g

- Protein: 28g

## *TURKEY LASAGNA*

- Prep Time: 30 min

- Total Time: 4 hr.

- Servings: 8

**Ingredients:**

- ✓ 3/4 pound Italian seasoned ground turkey breast

- ✓ 8 tbsp. chopped onion

- ✓ 2 finely chopped cloves garlic,

- ✓ 45 ounces tomato sauce (no salt added)

- ✓ 2 tsp dried basil leaves

- ✓ 1 1/2 tsp Italian seasoning

- ✓ 1/2 tsp salt

- ✓ 9 ounces frozen spinach

- ✓ 15 ounces part-skim ricotta cheese

- ✓ 16 tbsp. Parmesan cheese (grated)

- ✓ 2 cups mozzarella cheese (reduced-fat, shredded)

- ✓ 1 disposable plastic slow cooker liner

- ✓ 15 uncooked lasagna noodles

Directions:

1. Transfer the turkey and the onion in a skillet (10-inch) and cook for 7-8 minutes over medium heat. Stir from time to time.

2. Make sure the sausage is no longer pink before stopping the cooking process. Add garlic, stir and cook for 1 minute.

3. Drain, add basil, tomato sauce, Italian seasoning, salt and stir. Set aside.

4. The following ingredients will be mixed in a different bowl: ricotta cheese, spinach, 16 tbsp. mozzarella cheese and Parmesan cheese, as well.

5. The remaining mozzarella cheese will be refrigerated while this lasagna cooks.

6. The slow cooker (5-quart) will be lined with plastic liner. 1 1/3 cups of the above mentioned mixture will be spooned into the bottom of the slow cooker.

7. Make sure the sauce is evenly spread. Layer 5 lasagna noodles (if they don't fit well, you can break them). Spread with half the cheese mixture. Repeat this layering one time.

8. The remaining 5 noodles will be will be placed over the previous layers. Top remaining noodles with remaining sauce mixture, too.

9. The noodles should be completely covered by the sauce.

10. After covering the slow cooker, set the heat on Low and cook for 4 hours.

11. Turn off the slow cooker, spread the remaining mozzarella cheese over the last layers of noodles and sauce.

12. Cover the slow cooker and wait 10 minutes for the cheese to melt. Uncover the slow cooker and let stand for another 10 minutes.

13. The lasagna will be transferred onto a cutting board.

**Nutrition Information:**

- Calories: 490

- Total Fat: 14g

- Cholesterol: 60mg

- Sodium: 700mg

- Total Carbohydrate: 53g

- Sugars: 9g

- Protein: 38g

## ITALIAN TURKEY SAUSAGE CASSEROLE

- Prep Time: 35 min

- Total Time: 4 hr.

- Servings: 8

## Ingredients:

- ✓ 1 pound sweet Italian turkey sausage (casings will be removed)

- ✓ 1/2 pound lean ground turkey

- ✓ 8 ounces refrigerated onion

- ✓ 2 tbsp. garlic (finely chopped)

- ✓ 1 cup red wine (dry)

- ✓ 29-30 ounces diced tomatoes with basil, garlic and oregano

- ✓ 15 ounces Italian-style tomato sauce

- ✓ 6 ounces organic tomato paste

- ✓ 1 tsp sugar

- ✓ 1 tsp marjoram leaves (dried)

- ✓ 1 tsp oregano leaves (dried)

- ✓ 1/2 tsp anchovy paste

- ✓ 16 ounces spaghetti

## Directions:

1. After heating over medium-high heat a nonstick skillet (12-inch), transfer the ground turkey and the turkey sausage inside.

2. Cook for 7-8 minutes, breaking up with spoon. Make sure the sausage is no longer pink before stopping this cooking process.

3. Onion and garlic will be added, as well. Continue cooking for another 5-6 minutes. Stir from time to time and pause the cooking process when tender.

4. Pour wine and continue the cooking process for another 5 minutes.

5. Grease a slow cooker (5-6 quart), using cooking spray. Transfer the turkey mixture into the slow cooker and add the remaining ingredients (except spaghetti), as well. Stir these ingredients together.

6. After covering the slow cooker, set the heat on Low and cook for 4 hours. Stop the cooking process when the sauce is thickened.

7. Before serving this dish cook the spaghetti by following the indications on the package.

**Nutrition Information:**

- Calories: 450

- Total Fat: 8g

- Sodium: 1160mg

- Total Carbohydrate: 68g

- Protein: 27g

## CHILE BLACK-EYED PEAS IN SLOW COOKER

- Prep Time: 15 min

- Total Time: 8 hr.

- Servings: 6

**Ingredients:**

- ✓ 3 cups fresh black-eyed peas (shelled)
- ✓ 2 cups chicken broth (reduced-sodium)
- ✓ 2 cups sweet onions (chopped)
- ✓ 2 tbsp. jalapeño chile (finely chopped)
- ✓ 1/2 tsp thyme leaves (dried)
- ✓ 1/4 tsp salt
- ✓ 1/4 tsp freshly ground pepper
- ✓ 4 finely chopped cloves garlic
- ✓ 1 bay leaf (dried)
- ✓ 1 turkey leg (smoked)
- ✓ Red pepper sauce

**Directions:**

1. Stir together the all the ingredients in a greased slow-cooker (3 ½-quart).

2. Transfer the turkey leg in the slow cooker, too, placing it on top of the mixture.

3. After covering the slow cooker, set the heat on Low and cook for 8 hours.

4. The turkey leg will discarded, together with the bay leaf, too.

5. Use slotted spoon when serving peas.

**Nutrition Information:**

- Calories: 450

## *Slow Cook Italian Meatballs*

- Prep Time: 35 min

- Total Time: 4 hr.

- Servings: 12

**Ingredients:**

- ✓ 2 cups onions (finely diced)

- ✓ 1 tbsp. olive oil

- ✓ 1 pound extra-lean ground beef

- ✓ 320 ounces turkey Italian sausage

- ✓ 1 cup plain bread crumbs

- ✓ 8 tbsp. Parmesan cheese (grated)

- ✓ 2 slightly beaten eggs

- ✓ 8 tbsp. fat-free (skim) milk

- ✓ 1/2 tsp Italian seasoning

**Directions:**

1. The oven will be preheated to 400 degrees F/ 205 degrees C.

2. The onions and the oil will be microwaved on High for 4-5 minutes.

3. Stir from time to time and make sure the onions becomes soft. After dividing in half, set aside.

4. ½ of the onion mixture will be thoroughly mixed with the rest of meatball ingredients.

5. The newly resulted mixture will be shaped into multiple 1 ½ -inch meatballs. Transfer on ungreased pans (15x10x1-inch).

6. Bake until browned (16-18 minutes).

7. The remaining half of onion mixture will be mixed with the sauce ingredients in a greased slow cooker (6-quart). The meatballs will be stirred in sauce.

8. After covering the slow cooker, set the heat on Low and cook for 5-6 hours.

9. Make sure the meatballs are thoroughly cooked before ending the cooking process.

10. Serve with pasta and top with basil.


**Nutrition Information:**

- Calories: 250

- Total Fat: 10g

- Cholesterol: 85mg

- Sodium: 670mg

- Total Carbohydrate: 20g

- Sugars: 2g

- Protein: 20g

## *ITALIAN SAUSAGE AND STUFFED PEPPERS*

- Prep Time: 40 min
- Total Time: 4 hr.
- Servings: 4

**Ingredients:**

- ✓ 4 red, orange or yellow bell peppers (large size)
- ✓ 12 ounces sweet Italian turkey sausage
- ✓ 1/2 tsp red pepper flakes (crushed)
- ✓ 16 tbsp. onion (diced)
- ✓ 4 crushed cloves garlic
- ✓ 1 zucchini (small size; grated)
- ✓ 2 tbsp. tomato paste
- ✓ 1/2 tsp pepper
- ✓ 1/4 tsp salt
- ✓ 2 cups fresh baby spinach
- ✓ 12 tbsp. pearled farro (uncooked)
- ✓ 3 tbsp. fresh basil leaves (chopped)

✓ 1 tbsp. fresh oregano leaves (chopped)

✓ 12 tbsp. Italian cheese blend

**Directions:**

1. Prepare each bell pepper as follows: cut half inch off top stem end, discard membranes and seeds rinse these vegetables.

2. Stems will be removed and each bell pepper will be chopped from tops. You should obtain 1 ½ cups. Set aside.

3. The crushed red pepper and the sausage will be cooked for 9-10 minutes in a skillet (10-inch), over medium heat.

4. Stir from time to time and stop the cooking process when the sausage is no longer pink.

5. After draining, transfer to a large bowl and set aside.

6. Use the same skillet to cook and stir the onion and the over medium heat, for about 3 minutes.

7. Chopped bell pepper will be stirred in, as well, and the cooking process will be continued for another 2 minutes.

8. After adding zucchini, stir and cook for another 2 minutes. Add pepper, salt and tomato sauce and stir.

9. After stirring the spinach, too, continue to cook until wilted. Then, remove from heat.

10. Farro sausage will be transferred in bowl and mixed until it is well combined.

11. Onion mixture will be mixed in, too. 2 tbsp. of basil will be stirred in, together with 8 tbsp. shredded cheese and oregano. The farro mixture will be evenly divided among peppers.

12.   5 tbsp. water will be poured in a slow cooker (oval shape; 5-6 quart). Stuffed peppers will be transferred in the slow cooker and placed upright. They will lean against each other.

13.   After covering the slow cooker, set the heat on Low and cook for 4-5 hours. Make sure the faro and the peppers are tender before ending this cooking process.

14.   The remaining cheese will be spread over the peppers. Cover and wait 4-5 minutes, for the cheese to melt.

15.   Place the peppers on serving plates, using a slotted spoon. Sprinkle remaining basil over the peppers.

**Nutrition Information:**

- Calories: 420

- Total Fat: 14g

- Cholesterol: 65mg

- Sodium: 890mg

- Total Carbohydrate: 48g

- Sugars: 11g

- Protein: 25g

## *TURKEY BEAN CHILI SLOW COOK*

- Prep Time: 25 min

- Total Time: 8 hr.

- Servings: 8

## Ingredients:

- ✓ 2 pounds lean ground turkey

- ✓ 1 tbsp. olive oil

- ✓ 1 chopped onion (large)

- ✓ 1 poblano chile (medium size, seeded and chopped)

- ✓ 3 finely chopped cloves garlic

- ✓ 46-47 ounces great northern beans (drained)

- ✓ 3 cups chicken broth

- ✓ 9 ounces frozen shoe peg white corn (thawed)

- ✓ 2 tsp chili powder

- ✓ 2 tsp ground cumin

- ✓ 1 tsp oregano leaves (dried)

- ✓ 3/4 tsp pepper

- ✓ 1/2 tsp salt

- ✓ 8 tbsp. sour cream

- ✓ fresh cilantro

- ✓ Lime wedges

## Directions:

1. After heating over medium-high heat a nonstick skillet (12-inch), place the turkey inside and cook for 7-8 minutes.

2. Stir from time to time and stop the cooking process when the meat is no longer pink. Transfer the meat in a greased slow cooker (5-6 quart).

3. Heat the oil in the same skillet, over medium heat and cook the onion, garlic and chile for 5 minutes. Stir constantly and cook until the onion is tender. Transfer to slow cooker.

4. Transfer 1/3 of the beans and 1/3 chicken broth in a blender. After covering it blend for 20 seconds.

5. Make sure the mixture is smooth Transfer the mixture into slow cooker. Remaining 2/3 beans and chicken broth will be stirred in, too, along with the oregano, the corn, the chili powder, the cumin the pepper and the salt.

6. After covering the slow cooker, set the heat on Low and cook for 8 hours. Each serving will be topped with sour cream (1 tbsp.).

7. Serve this dish with lime wedges.

**Nutrition Information:**

- Calories: 370

- Total Fat: 12g

- Sodium: 1080mg

- Total Carbohydrate: 31g

# SLOW COOKER BEEF RECIPES

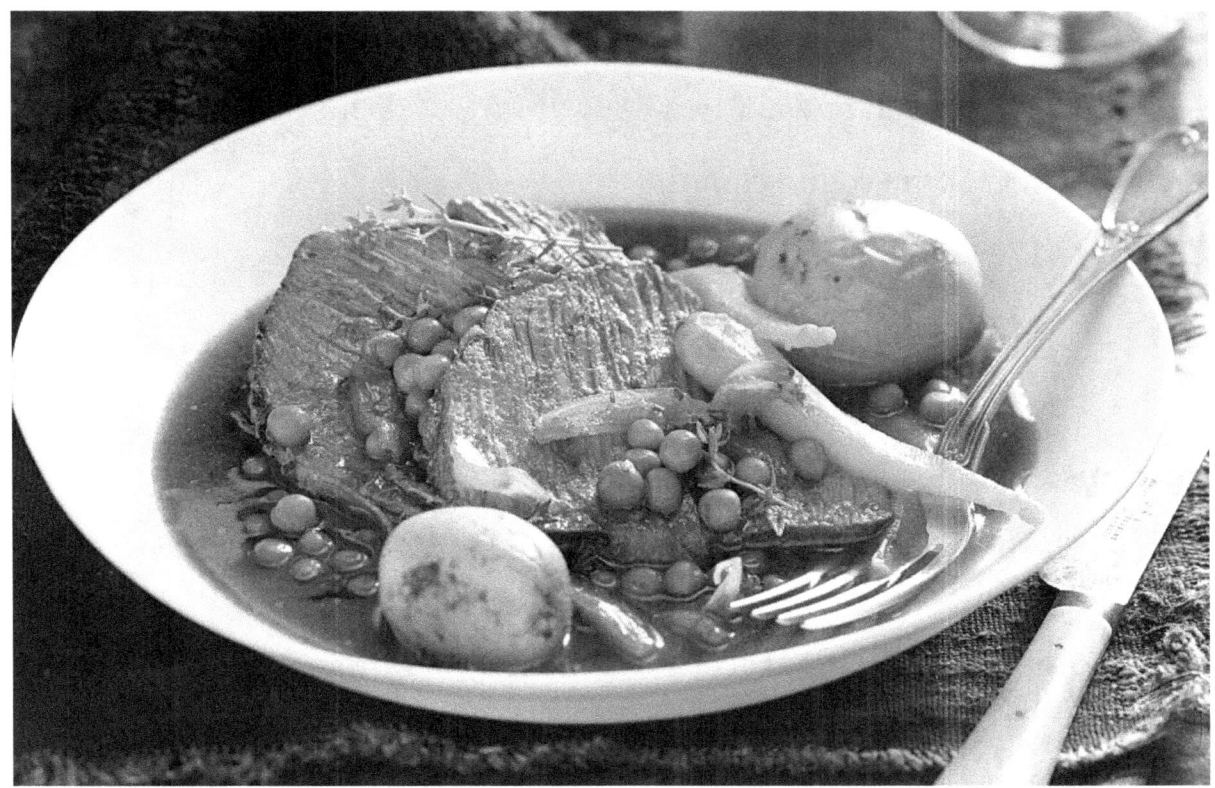

## CHILI BEAN AND TOMATO CON CARNE

- Prep Time: 20 min

- Total Time: 6 hr.

- Servings: 8

**Ingredients:**

- ✓ 2 lb. ground beef

- ✓ 1 onion, chopped (16 tbsps.)

- ✓ 2 chopped cloves garlic

- ✓ 28 ounces tomatoes (they will be diced and undrained)

- ✓ 16 ounces chili beans in sauce (undrained)

- ✓ 15 ounces tomato sauce
- ✓ 2 tbsp. chili powder
- ✓ 1 1/2 tsp ground cumin
- ✓ 1/2 tsp salt
- ✓ 1/2 tsp pepper

## Directions:

1. The beef and the onion will be cooked for 9-10 minutes over medium heat (use a 12-inch skillet for this purpose).

2. Stop the cooking process when the ground meat becomes brown. Don't forget to drain it.

3. The meat, the onion and all the other ingredients will be placed in a slow cooker

4. Mix the ingredients, cover them and cook for 7-8 hours over low heat.

## Nutrition Information:

- Calories: 300
- Fat: 13g
- Cholesterol: 70mg
- Total Carbohydrate: 20g
- Sugars: 7g
- Protein: 25g

# SALSA CHILI SLOW COOK

- Prep Time: 15 min

- Total Time: 8 hr.

- Servings: 6

## Ingredients:

- ✓ 1 lb. beef (ground)

- ✓ 1 chopped onion (8 tbsp.)

- ✓ 2 cups thick and chunky salsa

- ✓ 15 ounces tomato sauce

- ✓ 2 tsp chili powder
- ✓ ounces green chiles (chop them)

- ✓ 16 ounces pinto beans, (drain and rinse them)

- ✓ optional: cheddar cheese – it will be shredded

- ✓ optional: green onions – they will be sliced

## Directions:

1. The beef and the onion will be cooked over medium heat 9-10 minutes in a 10-inch skillet. Stir while cooking.

2. Stop the cooking process when the meat is cooked. Don't forget to drain.

3. The meat and the onion will be mixed with the other ingredients (except beans) in a slow cooker. Cover the slow cooker.

4. Cook for 9-10 hours on low heat.

5. Add beans and stir. Continue the cooking process for another 5 minutes.

6. Add cheese and onions, as well.

**Nutrition Information:**

- Calories: 290

- Fat: 9g

- Cholesterol: 45mg

- Total Carbohydrate: 31g

- Sugars: 7g

- Protein: 20g

## SLOW COOK BEEF ENCHILADA CASSEROLE

- Prep Time: 30 min

- Total Time: 5 hr.

- Servings: 6

**Ingredients:**

- ✓ 1 lb. beef (ground)

- ✓ 1 small onion, chopped (about 1/3 cup)

- ✓ 1 chopped clove garlic

- ✓ 11 ounces condensed cream of mushroom soup

- ✓ 4.5 ounces green chiles

- ✓ 10 ounces enchilada sauce

- ✓ 10 corn tortillas (6 inch)

- ✓ 12 ounces shredded Monterey Jack cheese

- ✓ Paprika

- ✓ fresh cilantro (chopped)


**Directions:**

1. The ground beef, the garlic and the onion will be placed in a skillet (10-inch). Cook over medium-high heat and stir constantly.

2. Stop the cooking process when the meat is cooked. Add soup and chiles and stir.

3. Grease a 3-4 quart slow-cooker and add 4 tbsp. enchilada sauce. Spread the sauce and layer 4 tortillas over it.

4. Add a third of the above mentioned meat mixture and spread it. Add 4 tbsp. sauce, again and 16 tbsp. cheese, as well.

5. The same layering will be done two times. You will use 3 tortillas, ½ of the remaining meat mixture.

6. Cheese and sauce will be added in each layer. Paprika will be spread over the top, too.

7. The slow cooker will be covered.

8. Cook for 5 – 5 ½ hours on low heat.

9. Cool for 5-10 minutes before serving. Cilantro will be added, as well (to taste).

## Nutrition Information:

- Calories: 500

- Fat: 31g

- Cholesterol: 100mg

- Total Carbohydrate: 27g

- Sugars: 3g

- Protein: 30g

# FLAVORFUL POT ROAST

- Prep Time: 25 min

- Total Time: 10 hr.

- Servings: 12

## Ingredients:

- ✓ 4lb beef chuck roast (boneless)

- ✓ 1 tbsp. oil (vegetable or olive oil)

- ✓ 1 tsp salt

✓ 1/2 tsp pepper

✓ 6 onions (slice them)

✓ 1 1/2 cups beef flavored broth

✓ 12 tbsp. beer

✓ 2 tbsp. brown sugar

✓ 3 tbsp. Dijon mustard

✓ 2 tbsp. cider vinegar

Directions:

1. Pour oil in a 10-inch skillet and heat it over medium heat. Before cooking the beef in the skillet, trim the excess fat.

2. Start the cooking process and continue for about 10 minutes. While cooking, turn the meat on all sides, so that it will brown on all sides. Add salt and pepper.

3. Transfer the beef in a large slow cooker and add the onions, as well.

4. The other ingredients will be added in the slow cooker, too. Cover the slow cooker and cook on low heat for 9-10 hours (if the slow cooker has just a heated base, follow the manufacturer's instructions in which regards the correct temperature setting).

5. Stop the cooking process when the meat becomes tender.

6. Use a slotted spoon to remove the meat and the onions from the slow cooker. The fat from the beef juices will be discarded (this is optional).

7. The meat can be served with juices.

## Nutrition Information:

- Calories: 330

- Total Fat: 19 g

- Cholesterol: 95 mg

- Total Carbohydrate: 9 g

- Protein: 32 g

# BEEF BURGUNDY SLOW COOK

- Prep Time: 30 min

- Total Time: 8 hr.

- Servings: 6

**Ingredients:**

- ✓ 1 tbsp. oil (vegetable/ canola)

- ✓ 2 1/2 lb. beef chuck roast (cut the meat into 1-inch cubes)

- ✓ 1/2 tsp salt

- ✓ 1/4 tsp pepper (black)

- ✓ 1 lb. carrots (use large carrots, peel them and cut into 1-inch pieces)

- ✓ 1 onion (medium, yellow onion; cut it into large pieces)

- ✓ 2 cloves garlic (chopped)

- ✓ 750 ml dry red wine (I would recommend Pinot Noir)

✓ 32 ounces beef flavored broth

✓ 1 tsp fresh thyme (chopped)

✓ bacon (5-7 slices, crisply cooked and crumbled)

✓ thyme leaves (optional)

## Directions:

1. Pour oil in a Dutch oven (7-quart) and heat it over (the temperature will be set on High). Use paper towels to pat meat dry.

2. Season it with salt and pepper and transfer the beef in the Dutch oven.

3. Cook for 5-6 minutes. Stop the cooking process when the caramelized crust forms on all sides of the meat. Then, place the meat on a plate.

4. Place the onion and the carrots in the Dutch oven and cook them for 4-5 minutes. Stop the cooking process when the vegetables become lightly browned.

5. Mic in garlic and cook for another minute. Stir in thyme, beef broth and wine. Make sure all elements are well blended.

6. The broth mixture will be transferred in a slow cooker (6-quart). Mix in bacon and beef, too.

7. Cover the slow cooker and cook for 8 hours (low heat). Stop the cooking process when the meat becomes tender.

8. Use the thyme springs to decorate the dish (this is optional, of course).

9. Freezer. Follow the directions as instructed through step 3. The beef will be transferred to gallon size freezer bag (plastic).

10. Seal the bag, making sure the excess air is removed. Repeat the same process for the broth mixture and bacon. The bags will be defrosted in the refrigerator overnight, before cooking.

11.  Transfer the ingredients in a slow cooker (6-quart) and cook for 8 hours (low heat). Use thyme to decorate.

**Nutrition Information:**

- Calories: 450

- Total Fat: 26g

- Cholesterol: 130mg

- Total Carbohydrate: 10g

- Sugars: 4g

- Protein: 39g

## *SLOW COOKER CARNE GUISADA*

- Prep Time: 5 min

- Total Time: 9 hr.

- Servings: 6

**Ingredients:**

- ✓ 2 lb. beef stew meat

- ✓ 28 ounces tomatoes, (they will be diced and undrained)

- ✓ 16 tbsp. onions (small and frozen onions)

- ✓ 1 tsp chili powder

- ✓ 1 ounce taco seasoning mix

✓ 15 ounces black beans (drained and rinsed)

✓ 11 ounces whole kernel corn mixed with red and green peppers (drained)

## Directions:

1. The onions, the meat, the chili powder and the tomatoes will be combined in a slow cooker with heating elements on the side and on the bottom of the cooker

2. Cover the mixture and cook for 10-11 hours on low heat.

3. The taco seasoning, the corn and the beans will be stirred in, too. Cook for 20-30 minutes on High. Stop the cooking process when thickened.

## Nutrition Information:

- Calories: 440

- Fat: 18 g

- Cholesterol: 95 mg

- Total Carbohydrate: 38 g

- Protein: 40 g

# DIJON MUSTARD AND BARBECUE BEEF SANDWICHES

- Prep Time: 20 min

- Total Time: 8 hr.

- Servings: 12

**Ingredients:**

- ✓ 3 lbs. beef chuck roast (boneless)
- ✓ 16 tbsp. barbecue sauce
- ✓ 8 tbsp. peach preserves (apricot preserves can be used, as well)
- ✓ 6tbsp green bell pepper (chopped)
- ✓ 1 tbsp. Dijon mustard
- ✓ 2 tsp brown sugar (packed)
- ✓ 1 sliced onion (use a small one)
- ✓ 12 kaiser or hamburger buns, split

**Directions:**

1. The beef will be cut into 4 pieces (first make sure you remove the excess fat).

2. The meat will be placed in a slow cooker with heating elements on the side and on the bottom of the cooker

3. All the ingredients (except the buns) will be mixed and poured over the meat.

4. Cover the slow cooker and cook for about 8 hours on low heat. Remove from heat when the beef becomes tender.

5. Transfer the meat to a cutting board and slice it (thin slices).

6. Return the beef to slow cooker, cover and cook for another half an hour. Stop the cooking process when the beef is hot.

7. The beef mixture will be used to fill the buns.

**Nutrition Information:**

- Calories: 440

# BEEF BRISKET SLOW COOK

- Prep Time: 10 min
- Total Time: 6 hr.
- Servings: 10

**Ingredients:**

- ✓ 3 tbsp. brown sugar (packed)
- ✓ 1 tbsp. and 1 1/2 tsp chipotle chili (powder)
- ✓ 2 tsp ground cumin
- ✓ 1 tsp celery salt
- ✓ 1 tsp( garlic powder)
- ✓ 1 tsp salt
- ✓ 1/2 tsp pepper
- ✓ 5 ounces beef brisket
- ✓ 1 and a half cups ketchup
- ✓ 4 tbsp. apple cider vinegar
- ✓ 4 tbsp. yellow onion (finely chopped)
- ✓ 1 tbsp. Worcestershire sauce

✓ 12 tbsp. low-sodium beef, chicken or vegetable broth or water

**Directions:**

1. Place the sugar, the cumin, the gallery powder in a small bowl. Mix in the chipotle chili powder, the salt, the pepper and the celery salt.

2. Grease a slow cooker and transfer the beef brisket inside. Add the above mentioned mixture in the slow cooker, too.

3. Mix the onion, half of the ketchup, the vinegar and the Worcestershire sauce in a different bowl. Pour this new mixture over the brisket, as well.

4. Cover the brisket and cook for 7-8 hours on low heat. Stop the cooking process when an inserted thermometer in the center of the meat will read 160 degrees F.

5. Remove the brisket from the slow cooker and place it on a cutting board, leaving it for 10 minutes.

6. Add the remaining ketchup to the sauce in the slow cooker. Mix well.

7. Slim slices of brisket will be cut and placed on the serving plate. Add sauce on the top of the brisket slices.

**Nutrition Information:**

- Calories: 430

## SLOW-COOKER BEEF STEW

- Prep Time: 20 min

- Total Time: 9 hr.

- Servings: 6

## Ingredients:

- ✓ 1 tbsp. vegetable oil

- ✓ 1 1/2 ounces beef stew meat (optional: cut the meat into bite-size pieces)

- ✓ 4 carrots (cut into thin slices, about a half inch)

- ✓ 3 red potatoes, (peel the potatoes and cut them into small cubes, about a half inch)

- ✓ 1 onion (cut the large onion into small pieces, about 1-inch)

- ✓ 1 medium stalk celery, cut into 1-inch pieces

- ✓ 1 ½ pint vegetable juice

- ✓ 3 tbsp. quick-cooking tapioca

- ✓ 1 tbsp. beef bouillon (granules)

- ✓ 2 tsp Worcestershire sauce

- ✓ a dash of pepper

## Directions:

1. Heat the oil over medium-high heat in a skillet. Place the beef into the skillet and cook for 5-6 minutes.

2. Stir constantly. Stop the cooking process when the meat is browned.

3. Grease a slow cooker (use cooking spray). Add the meat together with the rest of ingredients in the slow cooker.

4. Cover the slow cooker and cook for about 10 hours on low heat.

## Nutrition Information:

- Calories: 430

## SLOW-COOKER BEEF-SOUP

- Prep Time: 20 min
- Total Time: 8 hr.
- Servings: 6

**Ingredients:**

- ✓ 1 pound beef stew meat
- ✓ 1 large onion (chop the onion; you will need about 12 tbsp.)
- ✓ 1 large carrot (chop the carrot; you will need about 12 tbsp.)
- ✓ 1 medium stalk celery (chop the stalk celery; you will need about 8 tbsp.)
- ✓ 2 chopped cloves garlic
- ✓ 2 tsp sugar
- ✓ 15 ounces diced tomatoes (undrained)
- ✓ 21 ounces condensed beef consommé
- ✓ 1 tsp dried basil leaves
- ✓ 2 cups cheese-filled tortellini (frozen)
- ✓ 1 cup cut green beans (frozen)

Directions:

1. Add the following ingredients in a slow cooker: beef, onion, carrot, celery, garlic, sugar, tomatoes and beef.

2. Make sure the ingredients are placed in the slow cooker in the above mentioned order. Cover.

3. Cook on low heat for 9 hours.

4. Half an hour before the cooking process ends add the following ingredients: tortellini, green beans and basil.

5. Set the temperature to high, cover and cook for another half an hour. Stop the cooking process when the beans become tender.

**Nutrition Information:**

- Calories: 320

- Total Fat: 12g

- Cholesterol: 55mg

- Total Carbohydrate: 29g

- Sugars: 7g

- Protein: 25g

# BEEF AND POTATO CASSEROLE

- Prep Time: 15 min

- Total Time: 6 hr.

- Servings: 4

**Ingredients:**

- ✓ 1 pound lean ground beef
- ✓ 10-11 ounces cream of mushroom soup (condensed)
- ✓ 8 tbsp. milk
- ✓ 1/4 tsp pepper
- ✓ 2-3 ounces French-fried onions
- ✓ 4 cups frozen country-style shredded hash brown potatoes (from 30-oz bag)
- ✓ 12 ounces frozen cut green beans

**Directions:**

1. The lean ground beef will be cooked for about 7 minutes in a skillet, over medium-high heat.

2. Cook until the meat is brown. Add pepper, half of the onions and soup. Mix well.

3. Grease a slow cooker with cooking spray and layer the potatoes and the green beans inside. Add beef mixture, too. Cover.

4. Cook for about 7 hours over low heat.

5. Top with remaining onions.

**Nutrition Information:**

- Calories: 600
- Total Fat: 28g
- Cholesterol: 75mg

- Total Carbohydrate: 60g

- Sugars: 6g

- Protein: 27g

## STUFFED PEPPERS SLOW COOK

- Prep Time: 15 min

- Total Time: 6 hr.

- Servings: 6

**Ingredients:**

- ✓ 6 bell peppers (large ones)

- ✓ 1 1/2 pounds lean ground beef

- ✓ 2 tsp olive oil

- ✓ 4 tbsp. onion (chopped)

- ✓ 2 cloves garlic (chopped)

- ✓ 1 1/2 cups white rice (cooked)

- ✓ 1 tsp kosher salt

- ✓ 1/4 tsp black pepper

- ✓ 15 ounces tomato sauce

- ✓ 5 ounces Cheddar cheese (shredded)

**Directions:**

1. Prepare the peppers by removing ribs and seeds and trimming the tops of the bell peppers.

2. Transfer the meat in a large bowl.

3. Heat the oil olive in a skillet, over medium-high heat and add the onion. Stir occasionally and stop the cooking process when the onion becomes soft.

4. Add the garlic and continue cooking for another minute. Let the mixture cool.

5. Season the beef with salt and pepper and add the rice in the bowl, as well. Mix in the above mentioned onion mixture. Continue to mix until all ingredients are well blended.

6. The peppers will be stuffed with the beef mixture. Transfer the peppers into a slow cooker and add the tomato sauce, as well.

7. Cook the peppers for 6 hours over low heat. During the last half an hour of cooking spread cheese on top of the peppers.

**Nutrition Information:**

- Calories: 600

## *SLOW-COOKER BEEF STEW WITH MUSHROOMS*

- Prep Time: 20 min

- Total Time: 8 hr.

- Servings: 8

**Ingredients:**

- ✓ 12 new potatoes (they will be cut into fourths)

- ✓ 1 medium (chopped) onion

- ✓ 8 ounces baby-cut carrots (they must be ready-to-eat)

- ✓ 3.4 ounces fresh shiitake mushrooms, (the mushrooms must be sliced)

- ✓ 14.5 ounces diced tomatoes (organic and undrained)

- ✓ 1 can (10 1/2 oz.) condensed beef broth

- ✓ 8 tbsp. flour (all-purpose)

- ✓ 1 tbsp. Worcestershire sauce

- ✓ 1 tsp salt

- ✓ 1 tsp sugar

- ✓ 1 tsp marjoram leaves (dried)

- ✓ 1/4 tsp pepper

- ✓ 1 pound beef stew meat

**Directions:**

1. All ingredients (except the meat) will be mixed in a slow cooker with heating elements on the side and on the bottom of the cooker

2. For slow cookers with a single heated base, make sure you follow the manufacturer's instructions in which regards the ingredients layering and the cooking temperatures.

3. After mixing these ingredients, add the beef, too. Cover.

4. Cook for about 9 hours on low heat.

5. Before serving, don't forget to stir well.

## Nutrition Information:

- Calories: 230

- Total Fat: 7 g

- Cholesterol: 35 mg

- Total Carbohydrate: 29 g

- Protein: 16 g

## *FABULOUS MEATBALL SOUP*

- Prep Time: 10 min

- Total Time: 8 hr.

- Servings: 5

## Ingredients:

- ✓ 16 ounces frozen cooked Italian meatballs (thawed)

- ✓ 1 pint beef flavored broth

- ✓ 1 cup water

- ✓ 15 ounces diced tomatoes with basil, garlic and oregano, undrained

- ✓ 19 ounces cannellini beans, drained

- ✓ 6 tbsp. Parmesan cheese (shredded)

**Directions:**

1. All ingredients (except cheese) will be added and mixed in a slow cooker.

2. Cover the slow cooker and cook for 9-10 hours on low heat.

3. Add cheese on each serving.

**Nutrition Information:**

- Calories: 410

- Total Fat: 15g

- Saturated Fat: 6g

- Cholesterol: 100mg

- Total Carbohydrate: 38g

- Sugars: 8g

- Protein: 31g

# CONCLUSION

Slow Cooker mean to enhance your life, not burden it by cluttering up your counters and cupboards. This is one appliance that you can use daily, and I think that soon enough you will find yourself regularly depending on your multi-cooker to help you prepare delicious meals. Our recipes you will find wonderful flavor without sacrificing the integrity of healthy wholesome ingredients.

Thank you for getting my Slow Cooker Cookbook. I hope you enjoyed all these recipes as much as I have. I am always looking for feedback on how to improve, so if you have any questions, suggestions, or comments please Also, if you enjoyed the book would you consider leaving on honest review?

Thanks again, and have fun cooking!

**Maria Cook**